CW00449697

Other Books in *The Body & Soul* Series:

Sleep Tight

The Smarter Way To Sleep, Dreams, And Health
(Book 1)

∼

Also by Ian Breaker

Bored Panda, Banished!

5 Ways To Improve Life While At Home

Beat Your Weight Beat Your Fat

How To Lose Our Weight with Weight Loss Mastery

(Body & Soul Series, Book 2)

Ian Breaker

First Published by
Life

First Published January 2020 as
FAT: A Fix For Some Of Our Problems

Republished January 2020 as
FAT: Get Rid Of It

Republished June 2020 as
Beat Your Weight Beat Your Fat

www.beatyourfat.com

Part of the *Life Group*, visit us at:
www.lifegroup.life

Contents

Author Note

It's been suggested that some of the recommendations given here are too low in energy requirements to be gainful. Things such as slightly more heat production and excretion of wholegrains compared to refined grains, muscle retention, and getting up more often (such as during advert breaks). One remark is even that due to the thermic effect of food being such a low percentage of total daily energy requirements that having protein as a staple of our meals is little more than a paltry recommendation.

My initial response to these was dismissal as I found it difficult to believe they deserved to be taken seriously. However, I've now realised that this response lacks integrity. As such, I'll address it by saying that while any one specific recommendation might seem low in its energy requirements, it's the cumulative effect of all these little gains that results in something worth pursuing. Since the energy required to go from lean to overweight and then obese isn't all that much given a sufficient amount of time, every little counts.

By the same logic, while talking with the hands or fidgeting might not burn much energy when isolated to a single instance (and so therefore seems like it could hardly be notable in regards to our energy requirements), the sum total of all of our non-exercise activity accounts for a decent chunk of the energy we use in a day, therefore each part that makes up the whole *is* notable. In some cases, such as with the recommendation for minimal viable calorie reduction, the actual total you gain is more than the sum of its parts due to maintaining a higher metabolic rate (meaning you're simply using more energy by default). Likewise with protein; the benefits you gain from this nutrient are much more than just its thermic effect.

After all, the *real* energy balance equation is not:

calories in - calories out

But rather:

(calories eaten - calories not available) - (resting energy + cost of eating + non-exercise activity + physical activity + exercise activity)[1]

The point remains, if you want to lose weight you really ought to start taking command of your energy. Many of us are in the position we are due to being frivolous with our energy (mostly the intake of it because our output simply assists us with using what we've already taken in). Don't pass up on a gain (or loss) because it seems small in isolation; put it into the context of everything else.

This book covers practically every non-pharmacological thing that can assist you with both the input and output of your energy. It's not a sexy book. It's not a diet book. It is simply a distillation of everything I could think of that will both help and inform you on your fat loss journey wrapped around four main goals (in the belief that they will maximise adherence): to be sustainable, to be healthy, to be as non-restrictive as is feasible, and to be simple.

All the best,
Ian
Oct 2020

---

[1] This is RMR, TEE, NEAT, NEPA, and PA, each of which is highly variable. Each component of the in and out equation is also interdependent.

Beat Your Weight

to everyone

Introduction

Why is fat a problem? We're always being told to lose fat to improve health and that excess fat can cause problems, lead to various diseases and complications, and that we should really sort it out if we want to be healthy, but why? Why is 20% fat on a woman and 10% on a man considered slim and healthy, but yet add another 20% and they're now considered overly fat and unhealthy? What's wrong with being fat anyway?

Ignoring any of the mechanical reasons (and issues that result from it), the answer to this isn't so straight forward (nor is being overweight necessarily unhealthy, despite the stigma that surrounds it) because the level of fat that is unhealthy in one individual might be perfectly fine in another. Indeed, the problem is not fat per se as fat seldom kills us, but rather the various diseases that are linked to the fat that can pose a problem and potentially end up killing us.

As a matter of fact, it's not known what levels of fat are safe and what levels are unsafe for any particular person, nor is it completely known why fat can actually become a problem in the first place. All that's known is that, at some point, body fat becomes a health issue. There are three ideas (not mutually exclusive) as to why this is so:

The first idea is to do with the type of fat that accumulates, such that *visceral* fat is very much linked to these various health issues we keep hearing about. Things like insulin resistance (which is our cells not responding effectively to insulin so they don't take up glucose as readily), diabetes, heart disease, strokes and some cancers. Whereas *subcutaneous* fat is not linked to these health issues. Visceral fat is the fat that accumulates in the belly and a tight, somewhat hard belly is indicative of it. Subcutaneous fat is found all over the body (including the belly), and a softer, more wobbly belly is indicative of it. On this view, visceral fat is the problem and not just fat.

The second idea is based on the idea that when fat cells are full they appear to the body as damage, which results in inflammation, and so the body reacts accordingly. Inflammation is the body's first line of defence, but a state of chronic inflammation is not good for anything; it's been linked to cancer, depression, and Alzheimer's, and can lead to various complications throughout the body and with the organs.

The last idea is the idea of fat poisoning, called *lipotoxicity*. It's based on the idea that after our fat cells have reached their capacity and can't store anymore, any additional fat has to go somewhere else, but somewhere else are places it's not meant to go (like our liver and muscles). Fat in places it's not meant to go, especially in large amounts, can lead to a number of problems, often starting with insulin resistance. However, the amount of fat required for lipotoxicity to happen is different in different people because we all have a different safe level of fat storage; one person may be fine at 30% body fat when another is not fine at 25%. On this view, the health issue is not fat, but fat above our safe fat level.

I can imagine you're now wondering if there's any way of finding out how much fat we can personally store before it becomes a health issue? Well, unfortunately not. Currently there's no way to know if you're safe or unsafe at even slightly high body fat levels, but there are markers for health, such as cholesterol, blood pressure and blood sugar levels. But if we don't know when we're actually safe what are we to do? Well, ignoring getting checked up all the time, one way of ensuring our safety from any fat related issues is to not store excessive amounts of it in the first place.

But alas, the world has stored fat, lots of it, and there are more people dying today from the result of too many calories than too few. Quite shocking. Let it sink in a little. But what might be even more shocking is that those dying from the result of too many calories can also be malnourished.

This is certainly a problem, and there seems to be as many approaches these days to fixing the problem as there are people talking about it, and almost everywhere we turn there's someone new trying to sell us a fix. It's almost unfortunate that there's yet another person (me) who thinks they have something worth saying on the issue. But I think there's a hole, a hole that can be filled with a short and concise approach to a fix that is as non-restrictive and non-diet-like as possible (as well as covering what I see as the most egregious problem). A method that lies in the middle between the fad diets and waffle on the one side and the calculations and precision (and complication) on the other.

This way of proceeding won't suit everyone as there are real, tangible benefits to a weight loss approach that gives strict diet guidelines and a regime to stick to. The idea of not having to think and make decisions and so can just get on with dropping fat certainly has merit. But there are real problems with such an approach as well, the most dangerous being is that we seldom stick to it for good and so don't keep our fat off for good. After all, diets only work when we're on them, and we nearly always drop them over the longer term and so don't end up keeping that fat off.

On the other hand, the idea of not following a restricted food group diet and/or counting calories and macros has merit as well. We can just choose what we want from a wide selection of food sources and know how to eat whatever we want whilst aligning ourselves to whatever our current intentions are (e.g. losing fat). Suiting you, your lifestyle, and how you personally like to eat can have many benefits, most notably to me is a higher chance of sticking around over the long haul, i.e. your lifetime, because why would you stop a way of eating that you enjoy and is healthy?

There's actually another benefit to this way of thinking, which is that we're not having to 'go on' something, and remain on it, to keep a problem fixed. Instead, we're just moving forward with a different mindset and perspective, and don't have to then change our perspective to eat something different, we just eat something different whenever we want to. I find the analogy between a diet being a menu and a mindset and perspective being the entire kitchen rather apt. Knowing how to work the kitchen to fix our problem rather than being given only a select few items from within that kitchen certainly sounds like a better plan to me. As such, I won't be giving you a diet and this not a diet book.

But if we're not dieting how are we going to actually fix our fat problem? The same way diets do, because fat, in and of itself, is not such a complicated phenomenon. It's simply stored energy. And it's the result of more energy in than out. This isn't to say that various things don't contribute to excess energy and additional fat (like differing absorption in different people, sleep, or some of us storing fat more readily than others), it simply means that the ONLY way we can lose it is by doing the opposite. If we want to lose fat then we will have to consume less energy than we burn (or burn more energy than we consume— they're equivalent). We have to go into what's called a *calorie deficit*. There's no other way to do it (liposuction notwithstanding).

It's interesting as that last paragraph likely lost me favour with quite some number of people as they will consider what I've just said to be old-hat and that I've missed a memo, such that it's not actually energy balance at all but rather something else entirely, like some nuance of our biochemistry or a dysfunction of our energy storage systems or microbiome. This is unfortunate because despite various contributing factors to gaining fat (all of which do so by modifying calories in, out, or both, and we can give many of them a helping hand as we move along), any fat that we do actually gain is just stored energy that we haven't used. Such that it all began when we had some input (food and drink) and consumed a certain amount of energy, we then didn't burn the energy contained within that food and drink and so gained the energy equivalent as extra fat.

You may wonder why I've said something in the introduction of a book that I know will have lost me some percentage of readers, rather than wait until some later chapter to drop what some would consider to be not the most pertinent point to know when one wants to lose fat. I haven't gone mad (he says…), I've done it deliberately, and the reason is to let you know right at the start what central tenet underlies what I'm going to be saying, and we won't be using some other idea or some 'bio-hack' that promises us our goals by the grace of an angel.

We'll start with what I see as the problems, then move onto a fix, then the method that I advise you to use to implement said fix, and we'll finish with a discussion on how to not fail (the appendices are for ongoing reference and have some additional side information that you may find value in). So if you don't care for my theory then just jump straight to the fix as the fix will work regardless. The last chapter is the most important because any random tactic can be employed to lose fat. The trick is keeping it off. The human body loves fat. We gain it easily and readily and hold onto it greedily, and knowing how not to fail is of utmost importance because there's a high probability of failure if we don't do this right.

Push aside any impatience for pharmacological medicine to hopefully fix the problem. Food is medicine, and so our problems will be fixed by eating and drinking because we are what we eat and drink. We won't be fixing it by limiting food groups or starving ourselves, but rather eating all food groups in a way that aligns with fat loss. Limiting food groups isn't necessary because our problems aren't actually our food groups but rather our body and its energy regulation being led astray by an environment that's easy to get fat on and hard to lose it with.

The Problems

That environment is the problem, and we'll cover the food environment in this chapter as this is what I see as the main problem. For sure, there are other problems that contribute to gaining fat, such as a much lower energy expenditure for most people these days, and various genetic and biological influences that can help fat accumulate, but our energy expenditure has been getting incrementally lower for hundreds of years and yet our fat problem has come about only over the past few to several decades. New fat gaining genes also haven't swept through the human species recently and we've largely been the same for thousands of generations. This points to and emphasises the main problem being our food and our intake of it, not our genes or our energy expenditure.

Of course, this is not a new idea, and our environment has been touted as obesogenic for a while with our available food being one part of that obesogenic equation. Indeed, there is one particular proposed problem that I want to cover before we move onto what I see as the real problem. Before that though, let's just have a quick primer on the body and eating so we have a conceptual base going forward. We don't need to get into the weeds with this stuff so I'm going to keep it as simple and as concise as I am able.

GETTING FUEL

The body doesn't care what we're actually eating because as far as it's concerned it's all just sugar molecules, amino acids and fats, and what we eat and drink is broken down into these constituent components so our body can absorb and use them. Proteins are the amino acids. Carbohydrates are the sugar molecules. And fats are fats, both good and bad, in various forms.

Vitamins and minerals are used for myriad things to keep the body functioning well. Protein is used for building and maintaining tissue, hormones, and mediating bodily processes, among other things (our bodies are largely built from protein). Carbohydrates and fats are the primary source of fuel.

The fats, after being freed from the food, eventually get bundled back together into particles so they can travel around the system. They will find their way into the lymphatic system and into tissues and organs. Depending on the organ, the fatty acids will either be used for energy or stored in our fat cells. As an adult, we have a mostly fixed number of fats cells,[1] and we have billions of them all over the body. Some are under the skin (subcutaneous fat), some are in organs, some are in muscles, and some are around the organs of the abdomen (visceral fat).

The carbohydrates are handled differently. Carbohydrates are just sugar molecules linked together in various ways that are broken down into their constituent sugars and absorbed through the small intestine. There's 3 simple sugars: *glucose* (the body's first source of fuel), *fructose* and *galactose*.

The glucose component of the carbohydrate (or about 80% of it) is sent into the blood and begins circulating around the system (the other ~20% goes to or is taken up by the liver). High levels of glucose in the blood is toxic to the body, so in response to glucose our body immediately begins shuttling it off to various places. Some of the glucose is taken up by cells that need the fuel and some more is initially relinked together and stored as *glycogen*, the storage form of carbohydrate in our muscles and liver at about 2000 calories worth (the equivalent storage in a plant is *starch*, although it's a lot more dense than glycogen). If glycogen stores are full then excess glucose will be converted to fat and stored.

---

[1] ...which, as an aside, is why you shouldn't have liposuction performed because liposuction removes fat cells and not just the fat from inside the cells, meaning we'll have fewer cells available for our fat and therefore a lower safe level of fat storage.

This storage process is heavily controlled by *insulin*, and the end result is stable (and controlled) blood sugar levels that our body maintains for the purpose of providing immediate fuel to vital systems and maintaining consciousness.

And that, as they say, is that. I've omitted a bunch of stuff, of course, but that alone gives you the grounding you need to conceptually understand the root (and fix) for various things as we move along.

For now, one key point here is the part about our body's primary objective after eating being to get our blood sugar levels down by releasing insulin to shuttle the glucose to the cells that need it, and any left-over, unused and unneeded glucose gets shuttled into storage as expeditiously as possible, because herein lies a proposed problem that I want to cover first; the sugar and insulin problem.

A PROPOSED PROBLEM - SUGAR & INSULIN

This argument is somewhat multi-faceted and both can often be promoted as the cause of our woes. The argument is also said in various ways depending on who is saying it and what angle they decide to come from, but it basically goes like this (fair warning: there's a few technical terms in this section that may be new to you, which I hate doing, but stick with it. You don't have to remember them):

Our bodies mainly run on fat if we allow them to.[2] However, fat is stored as something called *triglycerides*,[3] and the body can't burn fat in the triglyceride state. To be able to burn the fat the body needs to break the triglycerides apart into its fatty acids. For this to happen our insulin levels need to drop because the enzyme that allows the fat to be broken apart[4] is inhibited by insulin. As such, since insulin controls both the storage of fat (by increasing after blood sugar increases and shuttling the glucose into storage) and inhibits the release of that fat for fuel (by inhibiting the enzyme that does it), insulin, and by extension, sugar, is the cause of obesity, and by implication, our health problems.

---

[2] Eating inhibits CPT-1 (*carnitine palmitoyltransferase*-1), which is an enzyme that allows fatty acids to pass into the part of a cell (mitochondrion) that generates usable energy (*adenosine triphosphate*, ATP). This makes glucose the primary fuel in the fed state, a condition that reverses in the unfed state, thus making fat the prominent during periods of fasting.

[3] 3 fat molecules, known as fatty acids, held together by another molecule, known as *glycerol*, hence *tri*-glycerides.

[4] *Hormone Sensitive Lipase* (HSL).

8

To some, it's not just sugar that's the problem but carbohydrates in general. We'll cover carbohydrates below when we discuss the actual problem, but since carbs are sugar, carbs are therefore the problem. Depending on what you've read previous to this you might have heard this said before. It's the main message behind the public advocacy of the ketogenic diet, for example.

The argument sounds reasonable, and I was partially sold on it myself for a while, but there's five problems with it.

First, there's a clue in the argument itself... insulin *inhibits* the freeing of fat for burning (known as *lipolysis*). It doesn't prevent it. Biochemists will tell you that the body works with something more akin to dimmer switches, not on/off switches; we can still burn fat in the presence of insulin because other hormones can also be at play that stimulate the freeing of fat, such as cortisol, epinephrine, glucagon, etc. These hormones are active together, so while insulin is inhibiting the freeing of fat, the others are *stimulating* it. Further, while insulin is promoting the storage of fat, other hormones are *inhibiting* the storage of fat (leptin, growth hormone, etc), so nothing is as clear as it first seems. It's worth remembering here that the human body is extremely complicated, so focusing on a single hormone and into a single biochemical pathway and presuming it tells us the full story is somewhat careless.

Second, why is it only sugar that's held up to account when protein can cause an insulin response as well? Some protein sources (e.g. whey protein drinks) are as insulinogenic as sugar itself. If we're going to say that sugar causes obesity due to insulin then we also have to explain why the argument doesn't hold for protein. One hypothesised answer is that protein stimulates the release of *glucagon*, which negates the effect of insulin. That may be the case but, once again, the human body is extremely complicated, and knowing how all of these hormones interact in different ways and at different levels in the presence of different foods taken in different amounts and at different rates is, in a word, *unknown*. Nutrition is not physics, and quantifying all the effects of an isolated nutrient in the human body is almost impossible for us. In a test tube, sure, but not in the body, not when not taken in isolation (which it seldom is), and certainly not for any particular individual since different people respond differently to certain foods; a cake to one person may spike their blood sugar through the roof but yet to another it may not (this is where the idea of *precision nutrition* is coming from, but that's likely years away). Since we don't know how all these hormones and metabolic processes act together the explanation proposed by the sugar-insulin model is therefore unreliable.

Third, giving people glucagon-like peptide 1 mimetics (such as liraglutide), which leads to an insulin release in the presence of elevated blood glucose, helps people lose weight and improves their health markers. If sugar causes elevated blood sugar that causes an insulin release that causes obesity, why does the insulin release in the presence of liraglutide do the opposite?

Fourth, eating *excess* carbohydrates stimulates *fibroblast growth factor-21* (FGF-21), which is a protein that improves blood sugar control, speeds up fat burning, slows down carb burning, and decreases appetite. This appears to be at odds to the sugar-insulin argument, because how do we explain it away when we're using the effect of carbs as a premise for obesity? As yet, there appears to be no proposed rebuttals.

Fifth, and that which looks to herald the sugar-insulin argument's departure, is that it basically contradicts *energy balance*.

ENERGY BALANCE

Energy balance is not complicated, but it's implications are all encompassing and it's never been found wanting. Before highlighting how the sugar-insulin argument basically contradicts it, allow me to elucidate a little on energy so you have a good grounding:

We must get the energy we need from that which we consume, and we're all familiar with this energy, we know it as *calorie*. A calorie is basically the energy contained within the chemical bonds of the food that we eat. (Recall above when I romped over how we get our fuel, with the body breaking apart what we eat into its constituent components. Well, that breaking apart of the foodstuffs into their components takes energy.[5] Your body then rearranges things and makes new bonds, which releases energy, and this becomes the calories, which are units of this energy. If the energy released is more than what it takes to break the bonds apart (which it always is), we gain a surplus).

Since our bodies use energy to perform all the tasks that it requires, if we

---

[5] E.g. glucose is a molecule of carbon, hydrogen, and oxygen atoms bonded together

don't have the energy we can't perform the task. And energy balance can be understood if we consider someone who requires, say, exactly 2000 calories a day to maintain their weight. That is, 2000 calories will neither allow this person to gain weight nor lose it. Now give this same person 1500 calories a day. This person is now in a 500 calorie deficit. This deficit *must* be accommodated for, irrespective of insulin (or other hormones), sugar, blood glucose levels, or any other biochemical term we care to drudge up, because they require 2000 calories and we've only given them 1500. They're missing 500 needed calories. Since we cannot breath in energy out of thin air this deficit of energy will have to be supplied from this person's storage of energy, i.e. their fat.

That, quite literally, is how energy balance works, and it breaks the sugar-insulin obesity argument (more formally known as the carbohydrate-insulin model of obesity, CIM) because if insulin caused obesity then a negative energy balance wouldn't result in fat loss in the presence of insulin, but yet it does, irrespective of the food eaten or the hormones that are present. Fat loss or gain *always* comes back to energy balance, and energy balance, achieved through calories-in calories-out, is actually something that can be manipulated in various ways to help us on our fat loss journey, and we'll be doing it all in what follows.

To be fair, the insulin argument also says that insulin makes you hungrier (due to high carbs/sugar in the diet) by emptying the bloodstream of glucose and fatty acids, thus signaling to your brain to eat, resulting in energy balance (due to the eating of carbs) routinely being tipped towards more calories-in than out. However (and the above argument on FGF-21 notwithstanding), insulin is thought to regulate appetite, not increase it, and the obese do not have lower levels of fatty acids in their bloodstream (sometimes they are even higher than normal), so part of this argument doesn't seem to hold up either. Of course, it's much easier to pick holes in an argument than it is to develop one, but the insulin argument just looks to have a few too many holes.

Regardless, we may think, sugar is bad through and through anyway, and we all know this, right?

SUGAR

Sugar has certainly gotten a bad rap nowadays, and part of the reason for this is that it's reached popular awareness that the sugar industry engaged in various unscrupulous tactics in order to sell more of their wares, but we need to be careful of the horn effect here; just because big business pushed their agenda for profit proves nothing except that they have a vested interest in pushing information that makes their product look good and their competitors bad. It says nothing about sugar itself, only about the companies that sell it.

However, don't think I'm saying that it's perfectly fine to stuff our faces with refined sugars and carbohydrates. I'm really not. Limiting these can be beneficial for various reasons, such as high sugar diets having been linked to inflammation (but then so have high fat diets as well as any other diet that results in excessive fat gain), and limiting them in a structured manner has been shown that it can help those with type 2 diabetes at reducing their insulin dependence, even to the point of pushing the diabetes into remission with some individuals.

Further, sugar is sweet to us (or at least the fructose molecule is), and humans love sweet stuff. Sweetness also activates the reward centre in the brain, which compels us to seek more of it, resulting in a somewhat reliable route to obesity. We can routinely gorge on as much sweet stuff as we like—and it's pretty much unlimited over the long term because there is theoretically no upper limit to the amount of fat that we can store—and we won't stop doing it because it gives us pleasure and therefore we don't want to.

For the record, I do understand the thoughts and concerns around sugar, and it certainly sounds like a bit of a rotten apple at times, irrespective of the insulin claims, but sugar is not 'bad'. And carbohydrates in general are also not 'bad'—they can actually be good, for various reasons, such as immune and cognitive function, and cortisol, testosterone and thyroid hormones.

If they were inherently bad I'd certainly be in trouble myself as I eat lots of fruit and veg, and I'm not shy with wholegrains either, but I am lean, and yet, as you can see, I subsist on a diet with lots of sugar. The problem with sugar is not sugar itself, but rather the *dosage* and *rate* of it, and the way we're consuming these carbohydrates in general is what can be ill-advised (refined carbs and free sugars), rather than carbohydrates and sugar being bad in general.

Sugar and carbohydrates certainly don't explain *why* it's so easy to get fat in the first place, nor why most of us are becoming so. For sure, if we couple these refined sugar and carbohydrate foods to the often high and easy calories associated with these foods this is surely partly to blame for our obesity and the difficulty we're facing with getting rid of it, especially considering that added sugar is everywhere and in most everything and often accompanied by lots of fat as well, so we need to fix it (and we will). But putting a lot (or all) of the blame at the feet of 'carbohydrates' is overly simplistic (and mistaken) as there are other problems with our food. Problems that look, almost inevitably, to lead us to becoming fatter. Carbohydrates have also been eaten for millennia and there's little that's inherently bad (save for tooth decay) or fattening about them.[6]

Our obesity problem is more complicated than this because we have also drastically changed *what* we are eating and drinking. Indeed, the most drastic way that our food environment has changed is by changing the rate at which this sugar enters our system, which can lead to many more calories consumed than we might otherwise would since it's so much easier and more pleasurable to do so. This has been done by the removal of *fibre*, not through the inclusion of sugar and carbohydrates.

THE REAL PROBLEM - FIBRE

It'd be appropriate here to explain *carbohydrates*, and in so doing we'll expose and illuminate the problem.

Carbohydrates are made up of sugar molecules and they've been given

---

[6] I can imagine that the low and no carb crowd will have a further problem with this. Glucose, they say, has inherent problems of its own and that it will damage you over time and so therefore should be restricted as well. Although it's true that the metabolism of glucose does have some potential issues (high triglycerides and aging of the body's proteins through tissue damage if your body is lacking a sufficient number of enzymes that eliminate free radicals) this is getting rid of the baby because it's got dirt on it, akin to never going swimming because some people drown. Eating lots of glucose that you don't need the energy of is certainly a recipe for fat gain, but the same can be said about any excess calories from any source. Only *after* we're developing a metabolic problem because of our fat does our general glucose consumption become a potential problem as well, just like overall calorie consumption does.

Moreover, carbohydrates appear to be more muscle/protein sparing than fat—that is, we won't lose as much muscle whilst we're losing weight, which is a good thing because we don't want to be losing muscle since it's good for us and aids fat loss directly (being more metabolic active than fat so burns more calories, even just sitting there).

three forms, *sugar*, *starch*, and *fibre*. These three forms are further bundled into two main classifications, *simple* and *complex*.

Simple: Simple carbohydrates refer to the sugar form, and there are many sugars, but only three simple ones (glucose, fructose and galactose). A simple carbohydrate refers to a sugar with a molecular structure of between one and two parts. For example, glucose, fructose or galactose, being singular molecules, are the simplest form of carbohydrate. *Sucrose* (table sugar) is two parts (glucose and fructose) and is therefore a simple carbohydrate. *Maltose* (the stuff that's in beer) is also two parts (both glucose), and so is also a simple carbohydrate. *Lactose* (milk sugar) is again a simple carbohydrate (glucose and galactose). Any more than two parts and the carbohydrate becomes a complex carbohydrate.

Food and drink containing simple carbohydrates are often remarked as containing 'free sugars', and our bodies love free sugars because they require little effort from our body to be absorbed (which makes the energy contained in them readily available). Simple carbs are absorbed rapidly (the quickest being liquid).

Complex: Complex carbohydrates are basically what the simple ones aren't, i.e. those with a molecular structure of more than two parts. As you would guess, the energy in complex carbohydrates isn't as readily available to the body as is the energy in simple carbs (mostly being due fibre content, particle size, and structural integrity).

Under the banner of complex carbohydrate is *starch* and *fibre*.

Starch: Starches are actually just sugar molecules linked together in long chains, but colloquially speaking things such as rice, bread, pasta, etc., are used to refer to a starch. They come in two forms. There's the *refined* form and the *wholegrain* form. Wholegrain is a descriptive term. It refers to cereals that have all of the layers of the grain still intact (the bran, which is high in fibre, the germ, and the centre/endosperm, which contains the fuel, in the form of starch). Wholegrains are, well, whole (save for the outer hull). Refined starches refer to starches that don't have all layers of the grain still intact, and have been refined to remove the outer layers and only keep the middle (the starch/sugar). As before, the simpler it is the more readily available the energy is to us—plus the body can end up excreting more of the wholegrains than the refined grains (e.g. course flour compared to refined flour), resulting in our bodies getting less overall energy from them in comparison to an equal amount of refined grain.

Fibre: This is the portion of carbohydrates that you cannot digest. It makes up the walls of the cells in the food that you eat (like vegetables and fruit), and the cells are where the sugar resides. Because the sugar molecules are contained within the cells then this, by default, slows down the rate at which the body can get at the energy and absorb it.

There are two basic types of fibre, *soluble* and *insoluble.*

Soluble fibre is so called because it dissolves in the gut, becoming a sticky glue-like substance that coats the walls of the gut and traps foodstuffs, further reducing the rate at which the energy can enter the bloodstream. It also provides nourishment to our good gut bacteria (more in the food appendix), which promotes the health of the host (that's you).

Insoluble fibre does not dissolve in the stomach, it absorbs water and bulks, resulting in a fuller feeling and therefore increased satiation. It aids in digestion and motility.

Reading that I can imagine you've already guessed at the problem I'm going to highlight. The problem is that these days much food is comprised mainly of quasi simple carbohydrates (refined) and fat and protein, with fibre and wholegrains seeming to be something of forgotten components. This is certainly the case with many pre-packaged and 'processed' foods,[7] which has done much to strip out any remnant of the fibre that might remain. Self-prepared food and meals can obviously be different, but even here the fibre seems to have taken a mostly back seat to the refined carbohydrates. This is unfortunate because fibre has several benefits.

As touched on above, when you eat a carbohydrate with fibre, say a price of fruit, the sugar is encased in the fibre and so the body can't get at these sugars quickly. The result, as with wholegrains compared to refined grains, after all work is told, is a greater production of heat, which is an increase to our calories out. To be explicit, non-refined or non-processed food takes 10%+ more energy

---

[7] Although I understand that 'processed' is somewhat ambiguous as the term can refer to nearly anything we do to food (cooking is a process after all), I'm using it as the term to describe the engineered side of our food. The side of food that most often results in it coming in a packet with a large ingredients list.

to process and utilise than do highly processed foods where much of it is simple and has smaller particle sizes. It's akin to the idea of eating a steak as a steak or grinding that steak into a mince—we'll get more calories out of the mince, and at a faster rate, than we will from it still being in the steak form because it's easier for our bodies to process the mince than it is the steak. A lot of our stuff these days doesn't even require much chewing (which takes energy, and therefore also increases our calories out), and we can almost close our mouths around it and swallow and have consistent and rapid calorie absorption.

However, the main problem with removing fibre is that we always end up with non-satiating, rapid, cheap, good tasting and moreish calories. So popular has this approach been to food preparation that it's now more expensive to buy something that hasn't been refined (which probably goes some way to explaining why obesity troubles the poorer members of society more so than the affluent).

Of course, you *could* get fat by eating too much fruit, such as pears and apples and dates and grapes (anything will make you fat if you eat enough of it), but you'll find it a lot more difficult compared to, for example, drinking the juice alone where it's easy to drift into the realm of very high calorie amounts. The same goes for all the other foods and drinks found on our shelves that are either refined and have no fibre and/or contain added sugars and fat.

Further, fibrous food has the effect of speeding up the passing of what you've eaten down into the small intestine, which then sends signals to your brain that you're full, i.e. that you're satiated and so won't want to continue to eat. Conversely, removing the fibre results in less overall satiation from our food because then the food doesn't have the same level of substance to begin with.

Moreover, removing fibre and substituting it with refined grains, free sugars and fat (and salt), which is what always happens, means that these things become very tasty to us, understandably leading to the drive to eat more of it, which makes fat gain reliable. They're quasi addictive and please us greatly. They don't satiate very well in the first place, and the satiation they do provide is gone in short order and so we're compelled to eat again sooner, which leads to us routinely going above our calorie maintenance levels. In effect, refined carbohydrates, no fibre, free sugars and fat makes us eat more by way of tasting good and making us hungry sooner.

The foods that result from all this processing are calorie dense good tasting little chunks of readily available calories. So dense are some of them that we can end up outstripping our calorie maintenance levels with just the addition of a few little goodies to our daily intake. For example, consider a requirement of 2000 calories a day for maintenance (a good enough metric for example). A doughnut containing ~200 calories, and they're tasty so we'll have 2. A single can of coke at ~150 calories. A single Mars bar at ~230. This is almost 900 calories, which is 45% our daily calorie allowance to not gain fat, and we haven't even eaten anything yet that we'd actually consider 'food'.

And it's not just the industry manufactured stuff that's like this as we can easily do it ourselves. For example, eating an apple means we're getting a decent amount of sugar, but if we turn that apple into juice then we're looking at around 5 apples to make even 250ml (depending on size of apples, of course, and how much of the pulp we decide to strain). And 250ml is somewhat small by my reckoning, a better quantity would be close to 500ml, which means we're now at 10 apples. Could you eat 10 apples in one sitting (and then still eat your evening meal)? I doubt it. But you'll do this without batting an eye with the juice. Just think of all the additional calories you're getting from this, calories that have next to no satiety value. Yes, a single smoothie a day can be considered one of our five a day, but so what? Just eat the fruit instead and don't drink your calories while pursuing fat loss, at least not regularly. Not being produced by industry doesn't mean it's not calorie dense and fattening.

That, fundamentally, is the problem with our food and the proximate cause of our fat.

THE 4-STEP PROCESS OF OBESITY

So here is the logical order as I see it:

1. Fibre is removed from our food, which exposes us to a food environment of readily available and super abundant calories; i.e. easy to come by, cheap, and with lots of free sugars and fat.

2. We're compelled to eat more than we require, for three reasons:

   • Because it's scrummy (and we all like scrummy things!)

- Our food choices don't adequately satiate us.
- This results in us feeling ravenous more often, compelling us to eat again.

3. ...but eating again isn't the actual problem. The problem is that once again we eat our current and readily available food environment, which is small packets of free sugars and fat at high calorie counts.

4. Steps 1–3 begin to repeat and then our problems begin.

THE MAIN TAKE AWAY

The main take away here is the extreme reduction in the amount of fibre encasing the sugars that we're eating. Stripping fibre means that the sugar that we are eating doesn't satiate us like it could. Or, said another way, removing fibre is a good way to make us eat more calories, in both amount with each sitting and more often. A reduction in fibre also brings with it an increase of sugar and fat into our diet and less bulk, which means more calories again. Removing fibre actually results in us getting more calories in general because the calories in our food and drink are so readily available.

• • •

It is often said, and it's true, that losing fat fixes all the health problems associated with obesity (inflammation, insulin resistance, cholesterol, etc.), so people are told to lose the fat to fix their health. But this largely sounds like it's their choice to be fat, and so to fix their health problems they just need to do something else. But being fat isn't a direct choice. Being fat is a *consequence* of interacting with our environment in a certain way.

The fix for this is *satiety*. Being satiated with our food choices means we don't keep eating and fueling the problem, and how we become satiated is by doing what we can to maximise our satiety levels. This isn't a tautology. It's simply pointing to *what we need to do*. Excess fat is basically due to being compelled to consume more energy than what we need because we're not satiated. This leads to more calories in than out. So what's the fix?

The Fix

Energy balance *always* dictates how much fat we will lose (or not lose), so ultimately the fix for our fat is necessarily a calorie deficit, and the two most popular camps around at the moment for giving us this appear to be the low (or no) carb crowd and the clean eating and plant based crowd. The low carb crowd extol the benefits of protein and fat and we can be somewhat confident that this is okay for us since we can point to the predominantly hunter tribes that look to have been doing it for millennia. The plant based crowd do the same with plants and we can likewise point to the predominately gatherer tribes for this. This looking to our ancestors for how we're meant to eat can appear to make a lot of sense because they're the environments that our current form evolved under so we adapted to them. No doubt. Both approaches do appear healthy and viable, and look like they could even save lives under specific circumstances, but the question of which one to pick or which one is best doesn't have to be an either/or answer. Our evolutionary history is not simple and there is no straightforward answer to what we're specifically adapted to; we are the result of both hunters and gatherers and are not directly descended from either one specifically. There is certainly no quintessential ancestor diet since any particular tribe would have eaten what they could get hold of.[1]

---

[1] Good data on their health is also lacking so we don't *really* know how they fared in their environment (and using modern-day foragers as proxies is just conjecture since extrapolating from these to the past is problematic, not least of which is that they've always been affected by modernity in some way).

Modern humans can eat, process and be perfectly fine with a multitude of foods because we evolved in a multitude of environments. We even have recent adaptions developed within the age of farming, such as tolerance of high starch diets and retaining the ability to process lactose into adulthood.

Even if there was a quintessential ancestor diet there is still no exact diet for everyone. People are different and they like different things, and it's perfectly okay to eat different things in pursuit of fat loss, which is why a non-restrictive and open diet can be important as it allows people to largely eat what and how they want (within reason, of course). This is why diets fail us after all. They restrict food groups for no necessary fat loss reason so we end up stopping the diet, eating the restricted foodstuffs again because we like them, and gaining back the fat because we never actually developed the knowledge of how to fix the problem in the first place. That said, diets do get some things right.

WHAT DIETS DO RIGHT

Successful diets work at losing fat since they wouldn't have achieved the label and status of diet if they didn't. This means they must have good points, and although I'm not going to suggest any specific diet as I consider it counter productive and unnecessary, this doesn't mean we have to ignore these good points. Nor should we. All successful diets do certain things right, and if we look at any successful (for losing fat) diet in the world we see that they all do certain things the same. They overlap, in effect, and the ways they overlap are the cause of their efficacy. Particular nuances of diets are just filler, both figuratively and literally, and are little more than a distraction.[2]

The first way they overlap, and the most important from a health, nutrition and fat loss stand-point, is that they all cut out (or heavily restrict) the *added sugar*. This is important because added sugar is just additional calories on top of whatever the food or drink is in the first place. The other way they overlap is that the foods they tell us to eat are *foods that result in satiation*. Few diets will advise us to eat something like a bowl of sugared flakes as a go-to meal, and nor should they, because all that this will do is result in either more hunger symptoms or more calories eaten due to lack of satiation.

---

[2] The ultimate reason for any success is a calorie deficit, of course, but I've taken that as a given so it's not included with the things that diets do right.

These two points aren't the only thing good about any particular diet either since diets can provide other benefits whilst we're in pursuit of fat loss. A plant based diet gets all the benefits of fibre and can allow us to eat whilst excluding animals products if that's important to us. Modified ketogenic diets that eat a fair amount of protein benefit from the satiation and thermogenesis (energy cost of processing) that protein delivers. Raw food diets get the additional benefit of being able to eat copious amounts and still being seemingly unable to maintain weight. Each diet often has a little extra due to its particular makeup, but fat loss is just fat loss, i.e. a calorie deficit.

The last thing that can be good about diets, and something that I mentioned in the introduction, is actually their restrictive nature. This might sound strange as I just said that this is why they fail, and it is, but some people benefit from the regimented nature of it, most notably if they enjoy the food groups they're restricted to. It gives an agreeable blueprint to follow. Whereas for other people, myself included, the heavy food choice restriction is counter productive and too difficult to stick to over the long term. I prefer to just do what I want with food for whatever current purpose I have of it.

A reasonable idea then is to take what diets do right and incorporate it into our own fix, but then forget about everything else since anything that isn't absolutely necessary has the potential to get in the way and cause problems down the line.

THE FIX

For the most part, there are really only two things required (in relation to food) to lose fat:

1) Restrict added sugar.

2) Eat satiating foods.

And there we are, how simple. Boring even. The difficulty with them is choosing to do them more times and often than choosing not to do them, and restricting added sugar in particular is not as easy as it sounds. This isn't to say you can't lose fat if you don't do them, but think what that would entail: You're eating non-satiating foods with added sugar, so you've had additional calories and are less full than you could have been. You also must remain in a calorie deficit to lose fat and so you can't just eat as much of this non-satiating sugary stuff as you'd like to, which means you're going to continually feel hungry whilst losing fat. Hunger is not a good feeling as we know, so if you go down the lasting hunger route it's likely you'll end up binge eating eventually and undoing all of your effort, maybe even quit it entirely until you're ready to give it another go. If instead you go down the route of actually satiating yourself with the non-satiating sugary stuff then you're just not going to lose fat because you're having too many calories.

On the other hand, doing just these two things means we've cut out lots of *additional* calories, plus we're satiated, so not hungry and therefore not continuing to consume more calories. These two points also come as a package and you shouldn't focus on only one of them exclusively, or think that only one of them is important. We can restrict added sugar and eat non-satiating so can end up eating a lot of calories anyway (for satiation purposes). Or vice versa, eating satiating foods with added sugar just means we're getting additional (pointless, and often invisible) calories on top of the existing foodstuffs.

As far as any priority goes, restricting added sugar is probably the most important thing to do and doing it will provide the most fat loss gains. There's a few reasons for this and first among them is that the calories you can drop by doing this can be pretty substantial since the majority of things in a packet have added sugar, sometimes lots, and it's often accompanied by more fat as well, which is even more calories. Reducing added sugar also reduces any insulin response, which can start to help you with any insulin resistance you may have. You will also find yourself automatically gravitating towards more satiating foodstuffs by default if you restrict added sugar. It's not a given as it's still possible to eat non-satiating foods even though we've avoided the added sugar, but it does point the way to the satiating foodstuffs.

Restricting added sugar also attenuates, and even prevents (over time), any of our sugar cravings, so we don't just keep stuffing our face with pointless calories, and it actually hard-limits our intake of simple and refined carbohydrates altogether, which, in effect, makes calories harder to come by. Removing the free sugars also means it removes the free fructose as well of course, so you won't be compelled to continue to eat more of it for the reward of sweetness.

Lastly, just to make it explicit, restricting added sugar puts a general cap on the foods that are making us fat in the first place (or at least making us fat easily and keeping us that way).

In regards to the satiation component there are two satiating foodstuffs I'm going to recommend here, *fibre* and *protein.*

Fibre: Fibre speeds the passing of the food into the small intestine so your brain gets the message that you're full sooner than it otherwise would. The insoluble component also absorbs water and bulks, increasing satiation levels. All sugars are encased, which results in trickling the energy into your system rather than spiking it. Fibre is also low calorie and has a somewhat high water content, which means we get fuller on less calories by default. Certain types of fibre also nourish our good gut bacteria (check food appendix), which results in us wanting and having cravings for these particular fibres (akin to the way regularly eating sugar causes cravings for sugar). The result is that this can eventually compel us to choose foods and snacks that are nutritious, fibrous, and filling, rather than sweet, moreish and fattening.

Protein: Protein takes quite some time to break down completely into its constituent components. It also finds its way further down the intestine before being fully absorbed and so fills us up for longer than most other foodstuffs. This workload also provides a secondary benefit, that of a high processing cost, meaning we use and burns a decent amount of energy to just digest, absorb and utilise it in the first place (you can notice this workload yourself in the warmth you get after eating).[3] It also stimulates the release of satiety hormones in the gut so you feel, well, satiated.

Two side benefits to higher protein in the diet is that it shifts the weight loss more into fat mass and away from lean mass (maximise this while dieting by aiming for 2.5–3.5g/kg of lean mass per day, spread out over your meals—increase the total by 1%+ per year after 30 to help attenuate the catabolic

---

[3] Depending on how much things are processed, which includes prepared and cooked, fibre and protein can cost up to about 30% of the calories consumed to actually digest them, compared to non-fibrous carbs at 5–10% and fat at a maximum of 3%. Generally, the more you process food the more calories become available. Available calories are also dependent on the individual eating them because people are different.

effects of aging[4]), and secondly is that it can mean we get higher levels of *tryptophan* (an amino acid), and higher tryptophan can mean higher serotonin, and higher serotonin can mean more happiness.

To sum up the benefits of these two steps I'll repeat that the foodstuffs of fibre and protein mean we'll often be getting lots of bulk and nutrients but at a lower overall calorie intake. They both have a high processing cost, so not only do we get the upfront benefits of them but we also get the hidden benefit of them burning a decent percentage of their own calories to just be processed in the first place. As such, if daily calorie consumption is kept constant then we can lose more fat, by default, simply by increasing the fibre and protein proportion of our meals than we would by increasing either fat or the other carbohydrate proportion of our meals.

Overall portion size is also important because we can get fat on anything if we eat enough it, and we'll cover that sort of stuff in the next chapter when we look at the method of all this, but the take home point here is to *restrict added sugar* and *aim for satiation*.

SATIATION

Put simply, satiation is being satisfied. However, animals appear to have nutrient specific appetites, and satisfying these appetites results in us feeling satisfied in the amount of food we've just eaten. The rub here though is that any particular nutrient specificity is particular to us, and so we have to find our own levels as they relate to us personally.

Before doing this, it's worth knowing a few things:

1. Energy intake largely hinges on satisfying our protein appetite, such that if we reduce protein we can end up increasing overall energy intake by way of the carbohydrates (everything grown by nature that we eat has protein in it).

2. Not satisfying our protein appetite in a meal leads to snack cravings, particularly cravings for savoury carbohydrates (and

---

[4] Lean mass is the result of your weight minus your fat mass, e.g. if you're 100kg and 30% body fat then your lean mass is 70kg.

if it comes in a packet it'll likely have added sugar, i.e. additional calories).

3. Highest energy intake is linked to meals low in protein and high in fat.

So given those points we can say that getting enough protein is important for satiation and can result in the lowest calorie intake since we don't then try and make up the difference with carbohydrates. The lower bound to prevent this is that the protein portion should be at least 20–25% of the energy value of the meal. This is no bad thing because protein is an excellent choice for fat loss aspirations: high digestive cost, high satiation level, aids in maintaining our metabolic rate, and helps us maintain lean body mass by shifting our weight loss more into our fat deposits rather than just overall bodyweight—all of which are good and are exactly what we want.

Nutrient specific appetites also inform us to be careful about cutting out the other macronutrients, as not satisfying one of our appetites is a sure way of making us want to eat something, so in the next chapter we'll be splitting our plates into percentages so as to give you a good starting point for this.[5]

We're getting into a bit of the method here but suffice it to say that you should feel free to experiment with your foodstuff portions in order to find your personal satiation levels because not everyone is the same with all food groups. Said another way, different people will find different amounts of different food groups satiating.

Since we're not restricting food groups this also means we're going to be eating starch and fat.

STARCH & FAT

To be fair, these are not exactly beneficial or good foodstuffs to use for pursuing fat loss, particularly refined starch. The reasons for this is that the starch is not very satiating (per calorie), they're both calorically dense (per given volume with the starch and per weight with the fat), and they're also very satisfying.

---

[5] Appetites are subjective. For instance, carbohydrate requirements seem to fall on a bell curve and some of us can cut them out almost entirely and be fine with it. Most of us cannot.

Basically, we like eating lots of them and we want to continue to eat lots of them, and so it's satisfying to put lots of both on our plates. The result though is that a high calorie intake is easy to achieve and therefore fat can be easy to gain.

Both of these foodstuffs can largely be considered an energy source, at least while dieting[6], and you should bulk on mostly fibre and protein as they are good for satiation and are nutritionally dense. You likely have plenty of energy in your fat stores to get on with so don't worry about not adding much additional energy onto your meals as the calories can add up fast, particularly from fat; it's easy to put 10–20g of fat on just a slice of bread or toast in the form of spread or butter, which gives us 90–180 additional calories, per slice![7]

Fat is 9 calories per gram, so 1kg of it is 9000 calories. It takes about 70 calories an hour to just sit and do nothing and about 100 calories an hour to stand and do nothing (although individual bodies are variable due to things such as lean mass, fat mass, age, and, generally speaking, the bigger a body is the more calories it burns). As such, many of us have months of stored energy that's just sitting there ready to be used.[8]

That said, don't be afraid of a bit of fat on your meat or drizzling some olive oil on your veg (although it's better to spray it for calorie purposes). And all of this doesn't mean you should cut either starch or fat out of your diet. What matters most is not whether you eat this stuff (you should eat them, and you *must* eat fat), but rather *how* you eat them, and that's the method.

---

[6] Yes, there's nutrients in starchy foods and fat is also an essential nutrient as the body can't make the essential fatty acids that it needs on its own so has to get them from our diet. Fat is used for various things, such as hormones, coating nerves, cell layers and helping us absorb vitamins (all but C and the B's, so be sure to eat fat with vitamin rich food), among other things, so don't go too low fat.

Try to focus your fat into mono-unsaturated and the omega-3's because, for the most part, we get plenty of omega-6 in our diet and very little omega-3. This situation has been linked to different things, such as inflammation as well as obesity in general, so consciously focusing our fat intake into mono-unsaturated and particularly omega-3 can be a reasonable pursuit.

As for starch, use predominantly wholegrain, and making it a *resistant starch* (heated and then allowed to cool, then ate cold or reheated) will increase satiation and produce short chain fatty acids in the gut, just like fibre, which appear to be beneficial for various reasons (decrease inflammation and risk of colon cancer, and promotion of a healthy gut).

[7] You can switch to plant based butter for (sometimes) lower calorie, e.g. *Becal* has 50% less fat.

[8] To be pedantic briefly for the sake of accuracy this isn't strictly correct since body fat is only about 87% lipid, so 1kg of it would be ~7800 calories, not 9000, but this shouldn't detract from the point being made.

The Method

So if being careful with added sugar (and fat) and predominately satiating by way of protein and fibre is the overall fix, how do we implement it? Well, this needs to be as simple as possible because the one dietary practice that's needed if we want to be successful over the long term is *consistency*. Doing something for a while and then stopping is why things fail. And consistency requires simplicity because then consistency becomes reliable and our nutrition is assured. Given the necessity of this, we won't be measuring our food or counting calories.[1]

GETTING OUR CALORIES

What we need to do is eat an amount of nutritionally dense, low calorie dense, and satiating foodstuffs to the tune of whatever is sufficient to satiate our hunger. We shouldn't be looking to lose fat by starving ourselves. We must eat, and eat quite a bit, too, since the best way of ensuring we keep the fat off is to actually lose it on the maximum amount of calories that we can still lose fat with.[2] This helps prevent the body going into its emergency mode where it

---

[1] But not counting calories doesn't mean that calories don't count. Calories always count.

[2] This further shifts the ratio of weight loss more towards fat and away from lean body mass.

drops our metabolic rate and ups our hunger in an attempt to gain back the fat we're losing (more on this next chapter).

Nutritionally dense, satiating foods are difficult to be consumed to the point of excess anyway since they are, well, satiating (and bulky), and excessive calorie consumption mostly comes from the foods and drinks that are dense with calories in the first place (added and free sugars and/or high fat). Outside of the calorie dense stuff, excessive calories can quite easily come from starch, particularly refined starch, and fatty meat if we're having a lot of protein.

Starch is actually something of a habit of many of us and we pile this stuff onto our plates like we're trying to feed The Ten Thousand or something. For example, how common is this look:

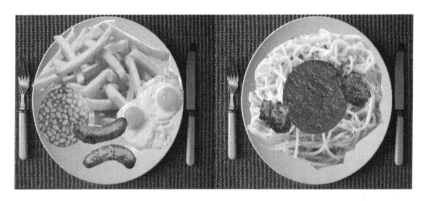

My graphic designing notwithstanding, it's pretty common. It's understandable why this is done as it's cheap bulk. True, but it's also a cheap and quick fat gain method. This is full-on carb loading, and it's absurd if you haven't got a requirement for high energy output (e.g. a sport). Further, you only ever need to do this if you don't have a lot of fat on you to begin with. If you do have a lot of fat on you then you just don't need to do stuff like this.

Instead of doing that do the following instead:

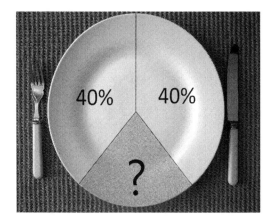

The percentages are the protein and fibre portions, and the question mark can be protein, fibre, starch, or a combination of them. As for fat, don't forget about it, but in most cases it's okay for the fat to be incidental since sufficient fat intake is easy to come by. If you believe you're having very low fat then eat it deliberately, maybe by way of the protein source or as something you deliberately add, like a bit of olive oil on the veg, etc.

You may not want to rush into this (more next chapter), but this is remarkably simple and easy and it actually removes the need to count calories. You can still count calories and/or macros if you wish, but only do it if you want to, not because you think you need to. What you need to do is separate your plate as above whilst not going crazy in the vertical dimension. Always drink before you eat and wait 20 minutes before having seconds. If you start to feel full before you've even stopped eating then you've already eaten more than necessary.

Just for the record, the above percentages shouldn't be used to argue for the validity in having some fast food burger or sub because the percentages turn out to be roughly the same. Ignoring the likely abundant fat and added sugar in that stuff, don't cheat yourself like this. The actual foodstuffs to be used for this are in the food appendix (there are many of them, and use it as an easy way of keeping you on the straight and narrow until you know what you're doing).

These percentages also aren't set in stone and we need to think about satiating our nutrient specific appetites. You should begin with experimentation in mind. For example, start with 40% protein, 40% starch, and 20% fibre and see how you get on.[3] I imagine you'll feel fine with this, and if so then keep increasing the fibre portion until it's 40% and the starch is 20%. If you're still fine then keep decreasing the starch portion and replace it with protein or fibre. If you're not fine with this and feel a little bloated or have unsettled digestion, then decrease the fibre and ideally replace with protein, but and/or starch as well. Either way, be sure to ease yourself into increasing your fibre amount. If you're not fine with 40% protein, 40% starch and 20% fibre, then try increasing the protein portion (fibre if it's comfortable to you) and ideally decrease the starch. If you find yourself needing more starch then an ideal type would be wholegrain, and resistant starch will slow its digestion and increase satiation. We're basically flirting around with our meals to see how high we can push the protein and fibre portions.

If you're already eating a decent amount of fibre then try going 50/50 with protein and fibre straight away (or even 60/40 fibre/protein). If you're full but feel like you're missing something then add a slice of bread to mop up the juice. If that works, then next time add some starch to your plate (unless you like bread and veg as much as I do then feel free to just keep having the bread instead).

The point is that you need to find out how high you can push the protein and fibre, but whatever you do don't fall back into piling your plate with a high percentage of starch. The goal is to be using protein and particularly fibre as much as possible to get satiation up as high as we can whilst using the minimal amount of calories. A side benefit to this is that the calorie amount from our meals is as low as possible so we can hopefully be more lax in other areas, giving us a buffer for other stuff.

You'll likely find it surprising as to how little calories you get from so much quantity once you start eating nutritionally dense, satiating foods and cutting out the free and added sugars (just try getting the calorie equivalent of a Big Mac Meal with chicken and veg—high calorie condiments and sauces notwithstanding). If you want some quantification for nutritionally dense, low calorie foods you could try the ANDI score.[4]

---

[3] I haven't made a mistake with these percentages. The reason for the decreased fibre and increased starch is that if you don't consume a lot of fibre already then jumping straight into consuming a lot can cause digestive discomfort. We should be looking to build fibre intake up over several days.

[4] https://www.drfuhrman.com/content-image.ashx?id=73gjzcgyvqi9qywfg7055r

You might not even be eating enough calories and would benefit from eating more (again, more on this in the next chapter). For now, just start splitting your plates and bowls up like the percentages above and eat an amount that's required to not still feel hungry.

Remember to drink before you eat (ideally water, plain or sparkling, but anything zero calorie). And remember to chew your food, as the faster you eat the more you will eat. Use the food appendix—all there can be recommended as a component to any of your meals.

HOW TO RESTRICT ADDED SUGAR

This is done by simply reading the ingredient list of foods and drinks and then not eating those with an added sugar component. Yep, you need to become one of those folks that reads the labels of their food. Starting with the liquids is a good plan since liquid sugar is one of the most fattening items due to an almost total lack of satiation that accompanies such a high calorie count. Another dangerous (for our waistline) arrangement is sugar and fat together since it's dense with calories but yet tastes wonderful, à la, desserts. The names of the dietary sugars are found in *Appendix 3 - Sugar Names.*

You'll likely find cutting out added sugar to be quite tricky, at least at first, and it's not because reading labels is difficult but rather because finding foods and drinks without added sugar sources can be difficult. If your general foodstuffs have much refinement then sugar is everywhere and in most everything you're having. You don't need to cut it all out mind you, and you shouldn't cut it all out immediately and straightaway as it'll just cause you to fail (next chapter). Further, once you've learned how to read nutrition labels (*Appendix 2*) you can choose to eat the sugar because you know the calories.

For now, just start becoming familiar with reading the ingredients and identifying the sugars (as well as fats[5]), and rethinking your meals with satiation and nutrition (i.e. the food appendix), and the above percentages in mind.

Maybe reading labels actually sounds boring to you but you need to know this stuff. I find it interesting, although maybe that's just me as I find that ev-

---

[5] Although if you find yourself gravitating towards fat rather than sugar you might get on well with a keto typed diet.

erything can be interesting given the right frame of mind. For example (and interestingly), why is so much sodium put into soft/fizzy drinks? I see two likely reasons: salt increases sweetness and it make us thirsty. The sugar masks the salt taste (it masks all of our tastes: sour, salty, bitter, savoury), and the additional caffeine makes it more addictive and use more of our water to process, making us even more thirsty. It's a 3-pronged gotcha ensuring that we want to drink more of it. Stay away!

If you find yourself craving sugary stuff and rich sauces then look into the substitutes to ensure you're getting the low calorie stuff. For a start, you can adopt sweeteners in place of sugar. These are hundreds of times sweeter than sugar so you're getting hundreds of times less quantity, so any caloric value is also going to be hundreds of times lower. If you're worried about any adverse health effects (which, to date, have really only been shown in rodents and petri dishes, and mostly at extreme doses), then worry about it again when you've got the big stuff in place and are doing everything else right that's assisting you with fat loss.[6] The effect of these is going to be minimal compared to the detrimental health effects of excessive fat accumulation—if you're one of the folks that has an adverse reaction, such as gastrointestinal distress from Aspartame, then switch to a different one. An often overlooked alternative is *Vitafibre*, which is a high fibre sweetener. Bear in mind that the packets of artificial sweeteners often have glucose and/or maltodextrin as filler, so care with the hidden calories that could accumulate here.

Another company that can assist you is *Walden Farms*, which has a selection of low calorie condiments, including barbecue sauce, salad dressings, and syrups. Low calorie jams/jellies also exist. Powdered peanut butter, such as *PB2* and *PBFit*, has most of the fat removed, thus resulting in much lower calories as well. Of course, not all condiments will need to be substituted because the calories are pretty low anyway, such as mustard and chilli sauces. Salt, of course, has no calories, and pepper is extremely low.

---

[6] This same argument applies to meal frequency/nutrient timing; it's largely a wash with regards to fat loss if you don't consistently have all your ducks in a row, and only then becomes something to consider (with the greater fat loss results coming from *changing* what you do, i.e. if you skip breakfast then eat it; if you eat breakfast then skip it. This is mostly likely due to you becoming more mindful of your eating).

Remember that *our taste buds are inducible* and over time *can be manip-ulated by our food choices*, so try and wean yourself off the abundant sweet stuff altogether so you aren't in danger of continually wanting to add additional calories to your food all the time (particularly important if you end up craving lots of additional sweet stuff after getting your first taste of it).

Keep in mind that we're cutting the added sugar because of the high amount of *additional calories*, not because "it's sugar", as not cutting these additional calories is one of those food choices that can actually make us fail at fat loss on its own because the calories can quickly become abundant and are accompanied with such little satiation, but there are things other than this that can make us fail, things that are more inherent to what it means to be human rather than something that comes from without.

How To Not Fail

Dieting has a low success rate, and the only two things known to be different between those that succeed and those that fail is consistency and the time taken to drop the fat. Those that succeed have found something that they can stick to and they progress forward at a slower pace and over a longer period than those who fail. Basically, the dieter who succeeds long term *enjoys what they eat* and has *patience.* They take things slow. Those that fail generally don't take things slow. They rush, and they don't have patience. They crash their calories because they want the fat gone as quickly as possible, quitting the method they used as soon as they've achieved their chosen weight because they never truly wanted to eat like that in the first place.

The problem with rushing and eating whatever is necessary to achieve fat loss with the intention of being fat free is that it doesn't work, and you're sacrificing your long term goal of being fat free for a short term goal of being fat free right now. Further, it can actually impair your metabolic rate to do this, impairment that appears cumulative on each iteration of you trying and failing, so if you've been going down this route for a while now and have become one of the untold number of yo-yo dieting victims then you need to stop it. This time we need to go slow and do it right.[1]

---

[1] An exception to this is if you're at some extreme body fat level (60%+). In such situations rapid loss might actually save your life. Bear in mind though that chemicals can be stored in our fat (known as persistent organic pollutants), in which case rapid weight loss would cause an abundance of these chemicals to be flooded into your system with untold consequences. These pollutants will be safer and less harmful when mostly locked away in our fat and allowed to trickle gradually into our bloodstream by losing fat slowly. All told, if you aren't in immediate danger from your fat levels then go slow!

Losing fat is never going to be easy however, and one of the difficulties with losing fat is that when we lose fat our body goes into a type of defensive mode where it increases appetite drive and becomes much more efficient at things it uses energy for. The more efficient it is with energy the more it has left to put back into our dwindling fat stores. It basically attempts to change our energy balance to at least bring us back to a maintenance level, and preferably into a calorie surplus.[2]

Let's elaborate on this a little so you can understand what's happening from a conceptual standpoint.

The following graphic represents calorie maintenance, such that the calories going in are equal to those going out.

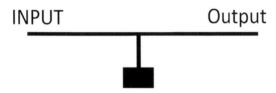

Now, when we either reduce our calorie intake and keep our output the same, or we up our output but keep intake the same, or we do both (reduce intake and up output), the scales now become this:

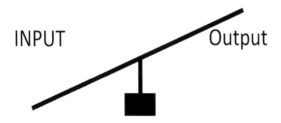

This is now a calorie deficit and we will be losing fat. However, if we put our maintenance level back in on top of this calorie deficit we can see that we've created a gap between the amount of calories required to maintain weight and the actual calories that we have going in:

---

[2] This is known as *metabolic adaptation*.

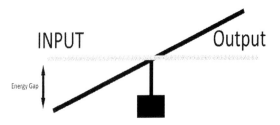

The size of the gap is the size of the calorie deficit, and when we start losing fat because of it the body's defensive mode kicks in, slowing down the rate of our fat loss. It slows down and saves energy on all of our outputs (anything that the body uses energy for[3]), particularly non-exercise activity (like fidgeting, talking with the hands, etc.), ups our appetite, and makes our fat cells more sensitive to insulin so they can fill up faster.[4] The whole thing is just a safety mechanism to protect us in times of famine, adapted due to the evolutionary fitness inherent in having such a mechanism.

So, with that description under our belt we can be explicit with the idea of having patience and going slow, and what we must do is try and make that energy gap between maintenance level and calorie deficit as small as possible whilst still losing fat because our defence system is proportional to the deficit, i.e. the harder we hit it the harder it hits back. And we can say that with the clarity of a picture, like so:

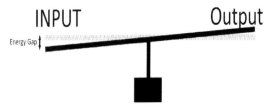

Doing the opposite and dropping a large amount of calories just makes the body more efficient with the calories it still has available, and we don't want

---

[3] At extreme levels it also shuts off reproduction and the immune system.

[4] You can also notice less of a warming effect from eating when this is happening because the body is processing things slower and so therefore not generating as much heat.

efficiency in fat loss, but rather inefficiency (a 10–20% calorie drop will likely work well). We can achieve inefficiency by eating more calories because the more we eat the less efficient and more wasteful our body is. Not only is this physiologically beneficial but perhaps just as importantly it's psychologically beneficial since deprivation based eating styles are unpleasant (and don't work long term). Patience gives us two things: not being deprived so much of the things we want to eat more of, and slowing down the body's defenses so it doesn't so readily sabotage us from the inside.

HOW TO GO SLOW

This is easier than it sounds and the way I suggest is to weigh yourself everyday, preferably in the morning after you've been to the bathroom and before you've eaten. Do this everyday of the week and take the average (as a percentage). A desirable speed of weight loss is *anything less than 1%* (less than 0.5% if you're already lean).[5]

That might sound a little complicated but it's not. Let's run through an imagined but workable example:

- Say you're 120kg when you start, and every day for the week (whilst dieting) you've been weighing yourself and the figures were 120, 119.8, 119.5, 119.7, 119.4, 119.3, 119.1.

- Add them all up and the total comes to 836.8. We then divide that by the total by number of days (7) to give us an average of 119.5.

- To find the percentage of weight we're losing we can divide our average weight by our original weight and multiply by 100, so (119.5 / 120) x 100 = 99.6%. This is our average weight as a percentage of our old weight (which was 100%).

We can see that 99.6% is under 1% less than 100% and therefore within the desirable rate to be losing weight. If we're losing weight faster than this then

---

[5] Although I don't much like the idea of weighing ourselves as it indicates weight loss rather than fat loss, what it does do is give us easy access to a figure that's often workable. A better indicator for fat loss is often hip/butt measurement (for women) and waist measurement (for men), or both. Even better is to weigh yourself everyday as explained above and also measure once a week. Don't bother looking in the mirror or taking photos until you're somewhat leaner since an untrained eye will struggle to see the changes, plus it can deflate you. If you can't resist visually inspecting then do it once a month, at most.

we should consider increasing our calories (or lower expenditure) as we may be losing too much muscle if we're going faster, and losing muscle isn't good since muscle is good for us and enhances our metabolism and weight loss ability.[6] If there are outliers in our weight during the week, such as maybe we binged or went out and drunk heavily etc., then take the median (the middle) value instead as this removes the outliers. Our weight can also fluctuate quite wildly day-to-day, so don't get too caught up with thinking about your fluctuations.[7] What we're looking for with our weight loss is a *downward trend over time*. We're not looking for spikes and crashes, but a consistent and gradual decline.

As mentioned, if we're losing weight faster than 1% a week then we might want to look into increasing our current calories since our defence system might be hitting us harder than necessary and/or we'll start losing muscle, and how we actually increase our calories largely depends on how we're currently dropping them, but in a nutshell we just need to eat or drink something that we've been neglecting. However, how we add calories is not as important as how we're dropping calories in the first place since slow weight loss requires a slow calorie reduction. The way we achieve a slow calorie reduction largely depends on what we're eating now, and to clarify this point there are as I see it two types of people that eat different types of foods, and so how they manipulate their calories will depend on which type they are.

THE TWO-TYPES

The two types are those who eat a lot of rubbish and those who don't eat a lot of rubbish. By rubbish I'm referring to things such as regular treats, like doughnuts and cakes, sweets, chocolate bars, crisps/chips (and dips), fry-ups, regular chips/fries, fast food, processed food, microwave ready meals, fizzy drinks, fruit juice, etc. This is the rubbish of the world. It's all very yummy. And it's easy to get fat on.

---

[6] There are those that don't necessarily have to go slow. These are the folks that are totally on board and committed to a marked change in their lifestyle. Such as maybe a light bulb went off in their head one morning and they dropped everything and started hitting the gym 5 days a week. Still not advisable but we can push through our body's defenses by being headstrong—energy is energy and our body isn't magic. After all, if we stop eating for long enough we don't stop losing weight, we die.

[7] During the first week of weight loss you'll also likely lose more than 1% as you'll lose a lot of water weight from tapping into your glycogen, which is 3 parts water to 1 part glucose.

The other group of people don't much partake in all this stuff. Sure, they may have some of them every now and then but they don't eat them regularly and seldom gorge on them.

Given these two types, how we should approach our diet depends on which type we are (check relevant section in references for eating disorders).

TAKE YOUR TIME IF YOU EAT RUBBISH

The first step here is to not initially focus on the fat but rather focus on the rubbish that you're eating. I understand that this might not sit well with you because it's the fat that you care about and want to get rid of, but just accept that the fat will go as surely as a child will eventually walk, and shift your actual goal to keeping the fat gone rather than getting rid of the fat right now, which means shifting your focus away from the fat and towards what's necessary on the way to getting rid of it for good (ongoing reduction of the rubbish).

After you've got it into your head that we're in this for the long haul and are going to do it right, the way to proceed is to *cut down gradually on the rubbish* over a protracted period of time. Slowly start swapping things over into the no added sugar, satiating, and nutritional categories. The goal is to get you out of the habit of having regular added sugar and refined foods and drinks and so eventually get you off the rubbish altogether (for the most part that is; we're allowed to treat ourselves after all).

Taking things slow just means you don't go cold turkey on the things that you like (and you certainly don't starve yourself, as mentioned). Going cold turkey just sets you up for failure as goodies are tasty and enjoyable and so knocking them all on the head immediately will be saddening and is very much a bad idea. Chip away at things and take moderate steps in cutting them out. Don't go from lots of junk food to zero junk food right now, today. That's the path to relapse and failure. You can have goodies, and you should have goodies if you've always been having them, you just can't overdo it. In particular, you just must *have less than you were previously* so that it starts the process off by pointing you in the right direction.

Specifics on taking it slow and with moderate steps would depend on what you're currently eating and drinking, but for example, if you're drinking several cans of coke a day then a moderate step could be to cut the quantity in half. A small step would be to cut a single can out and then cut another can out when you've got used to the reduced number. And *you must keep cutting* when you've got used to it—don't think you've succeeded when you've cut only a single can out. Instead, as soon as you've got comfortable with what you've already cut then you should be looking to cut again. If you have 3 sugars in tea then drop it to 2.5 sugars. Then when you've got used to that drop it down to 2. Then 1.5. Then 1. Then a half. Then knock it on the head (tea actually no longer tastes like tea when there's sugar in it). You do need to start reading labels so you're aware of all the added sugar you're having and remedy your intake of it *over the long term*. Change 10–20% of it at a time. Then, when you've got used to that (and not before), change another 10–20%.

Realistically, specific examples of what to cut could be as varied as there are people, but to monitor yourself, make a note of your food and drink choices throughout your days. To be fair, you know what's good and what's not, so go through the note and work out how to take a moderate step.

Of course, taking moderate steps means you're going to be moving forward slower, and the slower you go the longer it will take, which makes it somewhat of a balancing act between taking it slow enough to inhibit the body's defenses but fast enough to not annoy you with the time it's taking. It's not Sophie's choice though. Find your balance. It doesn't have to be so painful and unpleasant, so don't take things away that aren't doing you any damage. After all, no calories no problem; low calories low problem—zero calorie fizzy drinks, ~10 calorie whipped cream and syrup, etc.

I can imagine that this sounds pretty strange to you. I mean, have you just been told to eat sweets, and fast food, and drink coke if you want to lose fat? Well, not really, and there is certainly no chocolate or coke diet, at least not without explicit calorie counting with lots of hunger. Rather, what I've said is that if you currently eat these things then you don't want to stop eating these things immediately, or at least you don't want to go cold turkey on them. You need to reduce your intake of them slowly. Remember, job one is getting you off the rubbish. Job two, losing fat, will be coming along for the ride.

Actually, for another working example, let's say that you like your meals like one of the two plates from the previous chapter that were carb loading, such as the half plate of chips, sausage, egg, and baked beans, and we want to fix this with a moderate step with the goal of getting to the plate of the percentages instead. Well okay, we could progress a few ways here, but one way would be to have 40% protein (keep the sausages but fill the rest up with non-processed meat), have the question mark as fibrous vegetables and the baked beans and the other 40% as your chips. As a moderate step in the right direction *this is perfectly fine.* Progress forward from this point (when you're ready) by increasing the fibre content and decreasing your chips, and, at some point, swap the sausages (or even 1 at a time) over into non-processed meat sources. Lastly, take the beans off. The idea is to *keep nudging the bad stuff off* the plate little by little and replacing it with no added sugar, satiating and nutritional food. Moderate steps like this further helps us increase our fibre intake gradually.

However, with all that said, if you want to get more aggressive with cutting some things then you should do. Don't let the idea of moderation hold you up if you'd really prefer not to be moderate with something. A large part of the idea of moderation is to psychologically break you in to not having the sweet and moreish things so you don't miss them and become deflated and anxious about it. But if you decide one day that you're, for example, knocking fizzy drinks on the head altogether because you really don't want them in your life anymore then you should do so. Your compulsion and will to give them up will override any moderation benefits you'd get in reducing their intake over a longer period.

Regardless, whatever you do, you *must enjoy* what you eat, since if you don't enjoy your food it's never going to be something that you can stick to. If all you're doing is cutting out stuff you like and replacing it with stuff you don't like then this isn't going to be something that sits well with you for very long and you'll quit, probably falling back into old habits. Sure, you can deprive yourself briefly every now and then if you're looking for more rapid gains, but *don't do it long term.* As soon as you aren't enjoying the cut anymore then you've already been doing it too long.

For instance, I've recommended you heavily focus on protein and fibre to achieve fat loss, but what protein and fibre do you really like, and cooked in what way? Don't just eat dry chicken breast and piles of broccoli if it bores you. That's just… daft. I eat lots of broccoli, and sometimes chicken, as I very much like them, but I can't think why I'd consider siting down to a plate of chicken and broccoli alone. It sounds so boring to me. Satiation of your palate is equally as important as satiation of your stomach, even more so.

The Main Ingredients section of the food appendix has many foods, any of which you can use together cooked in multiple ways.

DON'T TAKE YOUR TIME IF YOU DON'T EAT RUBBISH

If you don't eat a lot of rubbish (and be sure you're being honest) but yet still have a decent amount of fat on you then there could be a few reasons for this, maybe only one, maybe two, maybe three, or maybe even all four.

The first reason for your fat could be that there is something in your diet giving you lots of easy calories. Excessive amounts of starch on your meals is one common and easy example. Starch is just energy, and if you're piling the starch on your plate akin to the two pictures in the previous chapter then this could be a cause of your fat. You can either burn energy or store it, and if you're not burning all this energy then you're gaining fat. Starch (and the more simple carbs) is actually the most variable foodstuff in regards to people's toleration of it as some people can eat a lot of it and some people can't. Cut your starch back to a maximum of 20% and fill the void with protein or fibre or both. *You don't need starch to bulk* (and you don't need to think about "carb loading" again unless you're lean) as you can bulk on protein and/or fibre just fine. The majority of my evening meals I just have a slice of bread for the starch. The rest is protein and fibre. Or even just fibre if I don't need the protein.

Another reason for your fat could be the added sugar. Added sugar is everywhere and you really must start reading labels to find it and cut it down since the calories can add up easily (refer to the Sugar Names appendix). We're blind to added sugar, such that we think we're only eating a slice of bread (and what's so bad about that?), but many add sugar (even some wholegrains do this, so be sure to read the label), and some add a lot of sugar, so we're eating the starch (which is sugar itself) for bulk and energy, but also eating the added sugar (which is just added calories) thrown in on the top. The only reason it's there is to add sweetness so it's more tasty to us so we eat more of it.[8] Added sugar is truly rife in our

---

[8] This isn't strictly true as not all things add the fructose but only the glucose, which isn't that sweet. The chips I had last night had added glucose. So I had glucose on top of glucose (energy on top of energy). Read those labels!

food, which makes additional, ready available calories also rife. Cut all added sugar that you're comfortable with. Anything in a packet is potentially rubbish (and the larger the ingredients list the more rubbish it is). The more you cut then the healthier and less fattening will be your overall food choices.

The third reason for your fat could be the holidays (or just the weekends in general). The majority of people will gain a bit of fat over the holidays, and this is fine, but the problem is that we don't take it off throughout the year, so the next year's holidays roll by and we've once again put a bit more fat on. If we do this every year and fast forward 10 years we've got 15kg of the stuff just sitting there not moving. Don't be fooled, you can put a lot of fat on over the holidays. You can also put a lot of fat on in a single day. Even with a single meal. To counteract this, first, be sensible over the holidays (and the weekends). Second, cut down on your starch and added sugar. If you're sure you're eating well (and being honest with yourself) and cannot understand why you're not dropping fat then you either need to cut your calories somehow (because if fat isn't moving then by definition alone you're not in a calorie deficit) and/or start exercising by involving yourself in something physical that you enjoy.

The final reason for your fat could be *lack of consistency* with eating well. You do well for a day, or two, or three, maybe even a week, but then you stuff your face with lots of rubbish and skyrocket your calories up into the multiple thousands, undoing all of your previous hard work. We'll talk more about this as we go, but *consistency is key!*

Some time after we've been refining our diet on an ongoing basis and are largely sensible with knocking the majority of the rubbish on the head, there will come a time when we are no longer able to continue to lose fat like we have been doing. We haven't upped our calories or reduced our energy expenditure but yet for some reason we've stagnated and don't seem to be making any more progress.

STAGNATION

Basically, at this point, you've plateaued, and your metabolic rate has equalised to your energy intake (as well as burning less calories because you're lighter), that you're back to maintenance, even though you're still on the same calories that you've been losing fat with. To continue to drop fat when you've stagnated you must up your output or again reduce calories (or both). Just view it as a sticking point, or a wall, that you must push through.

Stagnation in fat loss is very likely, but think about what we've done to make our transition through this as easy as possible: We've reduced calories-in by a minimal amount that we're still able to lose fat with, so when we hit a stagnation point we can just drop some more a lot easier than if we'd hammered the calories straight from the beginning. A couple of hundred calories will often be enough to push through a stagnation point (drop a doughnut, or the biscuits, or the generous servings of ketchup or mayonnaise. Go for a walk).

Compare this to a diet that drops calories with an intense calorie deficit so we can rid the fat fast. Pushing through stagnation on such a diet is tricky because we hit the calories so hard in the beginning. Moreover, if we do actually drop more calories then we're going to feel even more hungry than we have been up until now. Dogged, uncomfortable calorie restriction like this is actually setting us up nicely for hunger cravings and binge eating, which undoes our effort.

It's a terrible state of affairs really as most dieters will go down this latter route. We've been convinced that losing fat is the problem, and if only we'd buy that new diet or program that's been created or endorsed by the latest in a never ending line of pretty people who have been blessed with good genes and good looks we could rid our fat and look as good as they do. But the particular diet was never the problem. Nor was losing fat the real problem. The real problem is keeping it off.

I'm digressing, but as mentioned previously, anyone can employ a random tactic for losing fat. A diet of cigarettes, cocaine and coffee would work remarkably well. Even, less facetiously, if you only eat raw food you will lose fat, but the chance of you keeping that fat off for any extended period of time (3+ years) is approaching non-existent because it's a deprivation based eating style.

Tactics like that are less than worthless to us and we don't want to use them. We want strategy, and that strategy, as mentioned, is to go slow (less than 1% fat loss averaged over the week) and take moderate steps. Steps that align with where we eventually want to end up (restricted added sugar and good tasting, satiating, nutritional food).

How do you know if you've stagnated? At least 7 days that your weight hasn't moved. Maybe even 10–14. The reason for this is that a number of other things can cause our weight to appear to stagnate (fibre intake, sodium intake, water intake, activity levels, etc.), so leaving a decent amount of time allows things to normalise.

FIVE STEPS FOR SUCCESS

The habits you develop during fat loss will need to be maintained, so keep developing those good habits (reading labels, restricting added sugar, eating nutritional, enjoyable, and satiating foods) because they need to have become *an agreeable habit* or you'll fall back into your old-self, and, mostly likely, gain back your fat.

There are five further methods and habits that we can employ for assistance in our success, and not doing them actually increases failure rates:

- Exercising Control
- Being Mindful
- Keeping our Eye's On The Prize
- Having Support
- Exercise

Let's cover each in-turn:

EXERCISING CONTROL & THE POWER OF WILL

Our bodies are old and evolved in a time that was very physically demanding and replete with calorie shortages. A fitness adaption for such times is to crave energy rich foods and be lazy whenever possible to save the energy. All diets and nutrition programs can actually fail here because we don't really know how to fundamentally counter these once adaptive instincts for eating doughnuts and taking elevators. One way to offset these instincts though is by exercising our will and control over them.

Applying will power isn't always easy, and for sure there are hormonal and nutritional cues (fat, glucose, protein, insulin, etc,) making it even harder to apply our will to things. These cues circulate around our system and send signals to our brain, and our brain, in-turn, responds, and influences our next interaction with food. Moreover, the cues of the people who have a propensity for obesity make it so they are always slightly hungrier than the rest of us all the time. They're continually fighting their genetics, in the same way that many Labrador's are continually compelled to eat due to their cues and genetics. The difference between us and a Labrador is that we have the power to say no.

Now, although I'm not a proponent of libertarian free will, this doesn't mean we can't veto a decision with a free won't. We can compel ourselves to say no, but we can't decide whether or not we want to say yes. Don't try and attempt to change your mind so that it doesn't say this yes, it's *no* that you need to learn to say, in the same way that a nicotine addict learns to say no when they're quitting. They first developed that habit by saying yes, they then broke that habit by saying no for a sufficiently long enough amount of time.

A good way to begin with this is to monitor and say no to your impulse purchases, and then use the skill and discipline that we gain from this to aid us in saying no to our other impulses. Impulse purchases are everywhere, but let's think of the food environment.

You walk into a store. You have a list of things that you've previously decided that you need and so therefore intend to buy. The impulse purchase can raise its ugly head anywhere whilst we're in here, but consider the aisle on the way to the till. You know the score. You're standing in line, getting shuffled along like cattle, and with every shuffle you get a free look at something new, shiny and sweet, being nagged by the primitive part of your brain to just buy it and start munching. I could just tell you to walk on by and ignore the lot, but that's no doubt easier said than done for a lot of people, so here's a different approach: Forbid yourself from buying anything in the shop that wasn't on the list of your intended purchases when you walked in. Stick to your list. Adamantly. If you didn't remember it before you walked in then tough, you can't have it. If it's for someone else for some occasion that you forgot (valentines, birthday, anniversary, etc.) then sure, buy it, why not. But not for you. If it wasn't important enough to be thought of previously then it's not important enough now. This isn't punishment. It's habit forming. And it doesn't take long.

Another tried and true method of minimising the wish to impulse buy is to not go into the store (any store) hungry as you'll be compelled to buy more extraneous stuff. Sweet and fatty things look so much more tempting when we're hungry as it's how our brains work. Also, try not to shop when you're tired or stressed as your levels of ghrelin (the hunger hormone) are up and the brain's reward system will kick in for food more so than for other things.

Stopping the impulse buying is just a habit. That's all it is. And it can be developed pretty quickly. It's such a waste of money anyway, and you gain fat in the process. If money's tight you'll save a small fortune over the course of a year. Reinforce and speed up the habit building process by doing it with other things, too. Don't flick around window shopping on your tablet, then buying that nice pair of shoes that will go with that just remembered outfit of yours. Don't buy that adeptly marketed new toy that does basically the same as the previous one. And no, do not buy that Frisbee sized cookie because we get a second one for free. We do it for dopamine, that fleeting feeling of pleasure we experience when treating ourselves, or getting a Like on our latest Facebook selfie or macro dinner shot. Yes, acknowledging your own worth by treating yourself (or getting confirmation of your importance and interesting identity from others) is a good thing, but dropping the fat and fighting off the looming heart condition needs to become so much more important to you than a dopamine hit. So train your impulse restriction (it gets better with use). Make it good by learning to say no.

And stay vigilant. There's often a 2 for 1 right at the till, so even though you've survived the wall of shiny treats without being beaten you've still got to pay the fiddler and make your escape.

Stopping the impulse buying and sticking to your list are excellent types of external control over what you can and can't have, and if you do them for long enough they'll develop into a habit because habits start out as goal-directed behaviour, only developing into a habit when you've directed your behaviour for long enough.

You may not think much of the external control idea, but external controls work remarkably well (on adults as well as children, and we don't even question their validity with children). Think of external controls as akin to putting your child in the trolley seat so as to remove all the candy bars and sweets from their eyeline so you don't get nagged to buy them. The shops know that kids nagging their parents results in more impulse purchases. You know that out of sight out of mind and so the trolley chair can work like a charm. External controls can work like a charm in general. Use them to your advantage.

Another external control is to sort your kitchen out, which isn't a figurative statement. It's sorting your environment out and making it ineffectual for fat gain. *Put whole foods front and centre* and get rid of most of the rubbish (added sugar, non-nutritional, non-satiating foods), because if it's not there you can't readily eat it, and instead have to apply the effort necessary to go and get it (which you'll seldom do because you're intrinsically lazy like all of us). If you don't sort your kitchen out then you'll continue the same trend of adding to your fat because you'll be able to eat rubbish easily and whenever you want and you won't say no to the fattening foods as often as it needs to be said (don't remove everything though—take those moderate steps—but do hide it, as that way you don't have to continually say no the multiple times a day that you see it).

Remember to read the labels of things you have in your kitchen because fattening stuff can easily fly under the radar. A pretty common example of this, and one that could shift a bad meal a day into a good meal a day for you, are the ready porridge packets. You know, the portion sized, honey flavoured little droplets of goodness. It's easy to understand why they're popular as they're quick, convenient, easy, they taste good, and they look like decent food. Almost innocuous. But it's basically a dessert, and you should view them as such. Use wholegrain loose oats instead (put some real fruit in them for flavour. And/or Greek yoghurt if you like). The same goes for the yoghurt pots with the fruit at the bottom as they're designed in such a way that they look healthy and slimming. They're anything but healthy and slimming because you're eating syrup and sugar. A healthy alternative is to eat natural or Greek yoghurt instead (again, put some real fruit in for flavour. And/or oats). Low and no fat stuff can often be higher in calories because the drop in fat is accompanied by high added sugar to ensure it's still tasty to us (not always the case though, so read the label).

Either way and whatever you do, start sorting your kitchen out and getting rid of much of the stuff with high added sugar (meaning high and easy calories, and especially if it's a trigger food for you that you can't help binging on), since this can be another external control over what you can have. You're not starving yourself or going cold turkey remember, and lack of sugar doesn't mean it needs to be boring and dull, you're just further developing good habits during fat loss so they stick around with you after. The goal is to have, and also want, healthy, nutritious, satiating, *good tasting* food in our kitchen (despite minimal sugar). So start sorting your kitchen out over the next week or so. No rush. Look to the food appendix for lots of suitable things.

So that's two external controls that can aid us in staying on the straight and narrow (our note for things we're allowed to buy and a good looking kitchen). Another idea could be to reduce the size of our plates and glasses, both of which have substantially increased in size over the years (and more space mostly means we'll fill it up). Try also eating and drinking out of red containers.

Something else to keep an eye on and take a look at is our intrinsic laziness. Again, this is mostly a will-power, learning to say no thing. First, certainly say no to unnecessary elevators. I'm serious. Walk. Climb. Cycle. Run. Lift stuff. Move more. Whenever the opportunities present themselves. There are multiple reasons as to why this stuff is good for us so don't be shy of physical exertion. Doing stuff like this will likely have a greater effect on your daily calorie expenditure than a gym session will. Just getting up and walking about during the commercial breaks while watching television could end up burning a couple of hundred extra calories a day. Something as simple as climbing stairs instead of taking the elevators is a fantastically worthwhile thing to start doing; it burns additional calories, maintains and can develop lean tissue, and keeps stress on our frames, all of which are excellent health maintenance things for us to do throughout our entire lives. In particular, stressing our frame throughout life keeps our bones and skeleton strong into our later years so it doesn't crumble and start turning to dust so readily. More effective in our formative years (pre 25) but still beneficial all the way through. You'll be thankful for this when your bones are still strong and can still easily support you later in life. I'll cover exercise a little more under its own heading, but you're doing yourself no long term favours by avoiding the simple things that require decent physical effort.

BE MINDFUL

Another way that those who succeed at keeping their fat gone is that they are mindful of what they eat. They don't gorge blindly and habitually. They think. If they want that cookie they know they can have it, but they realise that they'll have to accommodate those calories into their day, and certainly not eat a packet of them and forget about it because a packet of cookies is comparable to a high calorie meal. You can eat the packet of cookies *or* you can have dinner. Every lick and bite of anything is going to contain calories, and these little things can add up over the course of a day.

With this in mind, here's a task you can either do now that will help you improve your food choices incrementally as you move forward, or start doing when you've been achieving decent fat loss so as to keep you on track. The idea is to make a note, on your phone, paper, wherever, of everything that passes through your lips throughout your days. This is both food and liquid. Make a note of *everything* as soon as you have it.

This gives us a record of the reality of our eating and drinking choices so it brings to light anywhere that we're tripping up. Be explicit if necessary. Don't skip on making the note thinking that you can just remember, as even though it might be possible to remember every little thing that you consume the chance of you forgetting something is pretty high. Plus we can often grab little snacks or drinks on the run without thinking about it or being lost in thought with something else—will you remember that habitual reach for the soft-mints or chocolates you continually have stashed in the car if you don't note it immediately? What about the habitual cup of tea with 3 sugars? Some fizzy drink or fruit juice would be another good example. These are important things to include but easy to overlook because they're habitual and often done subconsciously, so even though you might think you're on track and keeping on top of things you've actually forgotten a bunch of stuff that's throwing you off. Just deciding to make the note has the remarkable effect of you no longer consuming anything subconsciously and you catch it all.

Be sure to include the sauces and flavourings that you put on things as well as these can sometimes be even more important than the actual food itself, e.g. salad (which seems innocent) dressed with olive oil (important)—appendix 2 will give you assistance with this. But whatever you have, making a note of it can help us be more mindful of what we're eating, at least for a period when we're still needing some assistance.

EYES ON THE PRIZE

"Eyes on the prize" is an actual, psychological phenomenon, not just some self-help sound bite. It can help you achieve things faster and make the task at hand seem closer and easier. It can also work alongside a positive mindset, which achieves its results through the placebo effect (such as a drug easing symptoms when no actual drug was taken).

What is the prize? Well it's the dream that you want. A dream isn't the same thing as a goal. A goal would be to give up fizzy drinks. Or lose fat every month. The dream is what arrives sometime after you've achieved all those things, and it's important since "lose fat" and "keep it gone" is vague and you need something more explicit in mind. Maybe it's the figure? Maybe it's the health? Maybe it's to simply not die as young as you probably will? Whatever it is, a dream is not something that can happen later in life if we're lucky enough and life turns in our favour. It's something that we've become familiar with. Something that we know. Something that we continually work towards by achieving many small and readily achievable stepping-stone goals (stay off the fizzy drinks). It's something that we are keeping both eyes on. It's our finish line. Our target. And targets can be hit. Vague, wistful notions cannot. So get that idea, figure or health in your head and learn it. Keep your eyes on the prize.

HAVING SUPPORT

If you can (and if you're someone with which company helps you in this sort of thing), try and diet with someone else who wants to as well as this can give support and motivation. Generally, you'll want to choose someone who is positive and not negative (unless you respond to negative remarks better than positive, but few people do), such that the person you choose should tell you how well you're doing and how much fat you've lost, not highlight that you haven't hit your target yet and how much fat you've still got left to lose. They should be the type that tells you that the object is too far away not that your arms are too short. It'd also beneficial to be cognizant of the type of instruction that works best with you and choose your partner accordingly. For example, I respond very poorly to being told 'I should do this...' or 'I should do that...', I may even do the opposite just to push back against what I might see as an arrogant assertion. However, I respond very positively to statements such as 'have you tried this…' or 'have you tried that…'. Choose someone who's on the same wavelength as you.

Having a partner to diet with and give each other motivation can also help nicely with the next thing that can keep you on the straight and narrow: *exercise*.

EXERCISE

A full 70% of people who exercise after weight loss keep the weight lost, compared to only 30% of people who don't exercise after weight loss. The exercise you do should be anything that you enjoy and want to do regularly (aerobics, cardio, weights, a sport, dancing, walking, bike riding, swimming, etc). Exercising and developing lean tissue does a number of beneficial things. For example, exercising whilst pursuing weight loss can help prevent you losing muscle whilst you're losing fat (because losing weight means you could lose both), and this is a good thing because muscle is good for us—more lean tissue also means higher resting energy expenditure, which is a descriptive name and the largest chunk of our energy use. Basically, muscle burns more energy, even at rest.

Exercise also improves the metabolism by making the Krebs cycle (the using of stored energy) run faster. It creates new mitochondria (part of a cell that extracts energy from fuel), so energy is burned more efficiently and cleanly leading to more fat (and energy in general) being burned. It literally makes the heart stronger, and it increases circulatory health by enlarging very low-density lipoproteins (VLDLs).

It lowers your risk of many age related diseases and debilitations due to sarcopenia, osteoporosis, and atherosclerosis. It reduces the risk of Alzheimer's, cancer, and diabetes (can also assist in reversal of the latter). It helps protect us against the risk of a fall (especially notable for our later years).[9] It slows cellular senescence. It's a stress, depression and anxiety reducer. Over time, it's also an inflammation and blood pressure reducer. It's a happiness inducer. Psychologically, it can improve self-image, self-esteem, and confidence. It can even improve cognitive function and make us more productive.

It also looks like it can help with lowering the body fat set-point so you can stay leaner more easily. There are so many health benefits it's ridiculous.

---

[9] Couple with flexibility and balance training (or Tai Chi) for increased effectiveness.

Both young and old, exercise is amazing for us all.[10] Anyone who tells you it's only for 'vanity' is someone who seems to have missed every memo. Vanity will also seldom be a big enough driver to do it long term, due in part to the sheer amount of time it takes to see any of the imagined aesthetic results, most of which will be due to a lower body fat percentage, not because of working out—exercise because you love your body, not because you hate it.

You should start out easy if exercise is new to you. How easy? Easy! If it feels hard then it's too hard. You'll know when you're ready to progress forward with your intensity and/or duration because you'll feel yourself fitter. You also don't need to go crazy with the calorie intake after exercise as the calories you burn won't be all that much when starting out. The fitter you get the more energetic you become so the faster/harder/further you can go in the same time frame (which can result in a lot of calories being used), but when just starting out and/or you're not fit, the calories are low, so don't go thinking there's a void to fill.

Having a dieting partner who wants to exercise as well can be a huge boon as you can keep each other motivated, but even if you don't have a partner for this you should try and stick with the exercise anyway because being fit is actually more important for health than not being fat since health markers of those who exercise are higher than those who don't. But bear in mind that sedentary behaviour can also harm, so don't think that exercising gets you off the hook; make a conscious effort to move more, and move more often. Excluding fatigue and aggravating an injury or condition, there is no such thing as moving too much.

The last points to address, and something that could put a sticker in our progress, are environmental stresses.

ENVIRONMENTAL STRESSES

For the most part, the three worst offenders here for eating additional calories are tiredness, chronic stress (such as over a prognosis, not that you woke up a little late and are now in a rush), and boredom, and they can all compel you to eat (although this depends on the individual).

Tiredness can raise ghrelin levels (the hunger hormone), and this does exactly what it says on the tin: it makes us hungry. Cravings due to ghrelin are of-

---

[10] Exercise in water if your physicality hinders you (swim, yoga, Pilates, Tai Chi, etc), whether due to age, weight, pregnancy, or something else. Exercising in water is excellent for many reasons, including muscular, cardiovascular, and respiratory reasons, so it's worth considering regardless.

ten for high calorie and sugar loaded stuff, which I can personally attest to as if I'm tired I just want to eat sweet stuff and burgers, chips and cheese all day long.

Poor sleep could just be the result of various things leading up to your bedtime keeping you awake. Try doing the following at least 30 minutes before putting your head down:

- Switch your phone to airplane mode.
- Dull the blue light on your screens (or stop looking at them)
- Don't start a new project.
- Read something that makes you tired.
- If you keep a journal then write down the following day's tasks as this can be incorporated as a signal to your brain that this day is over.
- Dim your lights.

As for your bedroom itself, blacked out and cool is agreeable to most people for falling asleep, and when you're in bed stop thinking and just breathe instead.

As an aside, sleep also directly assists in the regulation and control of blood sugar by making your cells more sensitive to insulin (plus if you're sleeping you're not eating). Take a look at *Sleep Tight*, by Luna Green, if you're needing some assistance with your sleep.

Stress: Stress can cause weight loss. However, it can also cause weight gain as some people's reaction to stress is to eat. The mechanism mostly compels us to value calorically dense foods (chocolate cake, ice-cream, etc.) over other types as well, just like ghrelin, which makes matters worse. Not only can stress compel us to eat a whole bunch of calorie dense foods that we don't need, but stress can become unregulated where stress just breeds more stress, exacerbating the problem further (and is potentially dangerous, debilitating and even life threatening if we include the ongoing inflammatory responses).

Telling someone who's stressed to calm down might be like preaching to the converted, but here are some ways to reduce stress:

- Exercise
- Have a good sleep schedule
- Meditate
- Nature. Go spend some time in it (or find an artificial way to bring it into your life; smells, sounds, sights, etc).

- Play with/fuss your pets
- Quit nicotine
- Laugh. Laughter can heal, literally—try watching a bunch of funny movies, stand-ups, etc.

I touched on exercise above, but meditation would be an excellent approach to reducing stress long term, and it's not some new-age or mystic-guru rhetoric, so try not to think of it that way if that's the image that pops into your head. The meditation practice I'm thinking of is nothing more than a state of mindfulness, which is a quieting of the mind (rather than it being constantly chattering away). It can be done anywhere. In the quietness of your home or in the hustle and bustle of your commute. Eyes open or closed. You basically exist, peacefully, in the moment, with no thoughts buzzing around your mind, flirting in and out of consciousness, interfering with you experiencing the moment of now. Mindfulness also doesn't need to be something that you allot time to as it can be just done, e.g. you can be mindful having an orange (focus on the peeling and then the eating and the flavour). You will then also get the vitamin C from the orange, which can aid in lowering cortisol and in-turn your stress levels even further. Concentrate on breathing deeply; fill your lower lungs.

If you're not thinking you're not compounding your stress, as you will notice from your stress returning when you start thinking again. If all else fails, re-evaluate your decision to diet; it's probably not a good time to do it right now.

Boredom: Boredom can be bad for our weight because we'll often visit the fridge or cupboards when experiencing it looking for something to keep us entertained. As such, the cure is self-evident: change your current activity to something else that interests you. Above all, *keep busy*. This sounds trite, maybe even patronising, but be content with what you're doing and you won't resort to boredom eating. What you change to can be anything and doesn't necessarily have to be an activity of-sorts; changing the channel or watching a movie could alleviate your boredom. Read a book. Go for a walk. Phone someone for a chat, or go on social media and chat there. The point is, *change your current activity to something else,* as it's your current activity that's causing your boredom. If you're failing at alleviating your boredom and there's no stopping you from eating then *be sure to drink a big glass of water first,* and try and eat something high in fibre.

COMMITTED TO CONSISTENCY - *A Psychological Trick*

We all try and remain consistent to what we say because it results in a perception of honesty and integrity towards us. Businesses, organisations, and even governments use this often to elicit compliance, and you can take advantage of its power yourself. There's multiple ways to work this into our lives, but the way I suggest is to write down your fat loss goal on some cards and give those cards to all those people who you want the respect of. This will be an ally in keeping you on the straight and narrow because you won't want those people who you want the respect of to think ill of you. It can be a powerful trick, consider using it to your advantage.

IN CONCLUSION

1. We're looking for a small energy gap to attenuate the body's defenses and attenuate the loss of muscle (so a small calorie deficit).

2. Aim for a weight loss amount of less than 1% averaged over the week.

3. If you eat a lot of rubbish then focus first on getting rid of that rubbish a little bit at a time by nudging it off the menu and taking moderate steps into appropriate foods. Your fat loss will be joining you automatically in the process because small improvements, when done consistently, add up.

4. If you don't eat a lot of rubbish then cut your starch amount, cut added sugar, be mindful of the fat content of your food, be sensible over the holidays (including the weekends), and *be consistent*. Be physically active in something if you can.

5. Push through any stagnation by dropping some calories (couple of hundred should suffice), upping output (go for a walk), or both.

6. Seriously consider the five steps to success (exercising control, being mindful, keeping your eyes on the prize, having support and exercise) as your probability of failing skyrockets without them (particularly the first two and exercise).

Epilogue

THE ONLY DIET PLAN WORTH CONSIDERING

This might have seemed like a long road, and I don't want to diminish the importance in what you've done (or the hardship it took or is going to take) because losing fat is nothing if not a long process of continued effort, but to achieve your desired level of fat over the long term the road should remain easy to walk. Without wishing to push the metaphor too far, it should be laid smooth, exhibiting little resistance and with no potholes looking to trip you up. By this I mean that, once again, the method you are using for fat loss should be a method that you can stick to for good. It should be easy. It should not feel like work. It should not consist of boring foods that you don't like. You must like what you are doing because *you must be able to stick to it*. And that is the only diet plan worth considering: the one that you can stick to.

Sticking to it doesn't mean that you can do it for a year if you try hard enough. It means that you can do it easily and without hassle until the day that they finally put dirt on you. And it's called a nutrition plan, not a diet plan.

Don't underestimate this idea. If you can't stick to your eating plan and method then, well, you're going to come unstuck. So whilst I've given my recommendation on how to eat, based, in large part, on how I eat myself, this doesn't mean it's going to work for everyone and you should only adopt a method that works for you and your life because if you aren't (or can't be) consistent with your fat loss regimen then *it will not work*.

This method is predominately focused on protein and fibre (and being careful with and modifying your starch and fat portions) because they're excellent for fat loss (as well as maintenance) due to the aforementioned reasons. However, if this really doesn't sit well with you and you can't fathom out how to make agreeable meals and snacks from the protein and fibre sections of the appendix then, unfortunately, this method is not for you. It's not going to work if you don't like enough of the food items that I've recommended.

If you like one food group but not the other you could actually adopt a more focused diet. For example, if you like the idea of fibre but not protein then maybe a plant based diet would suit you better. Or if you like the protein and not the fibre then maybe a carnivore diet would work best. Or if you don't care for either then maybe even a Japanese diet, with its high carbs and low fat emphasis. I wouldn't feel comfortable recommending anything without fibre, but the choice is yours.

The point is, don't get stuck to some particular eating method and then become tribal, zealous or evangelical about it. They are all just tools, and tools are just there to be used in order to achieve a goal. Use the one (or ones) that sit well with you, that you like and enjoy, that are not difficult, and that you can stick to until the day that you die.

However, whatever method you adopt be sure to incorporate how not to fail with it. That chapter is not optional; do not approach your diet in a whimsical manner—treat it seriously. Don't become a recidivist by being blasé with your calorie restriction and then end up binging due to the deprivation, or lowering your metabolic rate to the point that you then have to exist on 1000 calories a day in order to not put the fat back on. You won't be enjoying life in this state. So don't go cold turkey. Don't rush. Aim for a consistent and gradual decline. *Have patience.*

PAYING THE PRICE

I find that achieving difficult things (like losing fat) often hinges on the idea of *paying the price*. We can fail to do things we want to do because we're not willing to pay the price for achieving them. Every thing we want to do has a cost associated with achieving it, and so every decision in life has a shadow partner, which is the cost and what we give up to achieve it. Even inaction has consequences. You cannot have it all, so don't even try. Things have to go. Give up the notion of being able to slim down and still gorge on sweets and treats in addition to inappropriate meals. Are you willing to pay this price? Don't give a knee-jerk reaction, have a think about it. Treats and goodies have to wait until we've taken care of the other necessary things, like losing fat, however long that may take. This is called delayed gratification, and it's a large indicator of success in doing anything. Learning it and applying it leads to tangible results.

If you're not willing to pay the price then give up now. Remember, we're changing for life. Life! So don't put yourself through it all if you're not ready to do it right now, whether mentally or otherwise. It's not that you can't do it, and we're not chasing rainbows here, but the cost of action has to be something you're willing to pay, and pay long term because for the love of your health you don't want to remain on the yo-yo dieting treadmill.

There's nothing wrong with not being willing to pay the price, and you certainly don't have to be slim, nor can everyone be slim because it might be just too difficult for them to maintain. But wherever you want to be, and wherever you comfortably can be, you need to be willing to pay the price for it, and you'll need to be willing to pay it at crunch time when there's a choice to be made. Some choices are easy and some difficult. Losing fat is difficult, so don't feel bad that it's difficult for you, too. It can even be painful. But this is just cost. And it is you who will need to pay this cost.

The cost can sometimes be emotional, say from set backs, which can lead to feelings of failure, depleting our emotional bank account. When that goes it feels like the cost immediately shoots through the roof and it's no longer a cost but a debt. Our will to continue collapses and we turn a blind eye with feigned nonchalance or, worse, pity. A trick is to know categorically that failing isn't failure (and what doesn't kill you could even make you stronger). It's only failure if you don't put yourself back on track, so always *try to go further than your last failing.* Acknowledge the knock but will yourself forwards anyway. Try and nurture urgency since urgency breeds seriousness and sets you up confidently to pay a price (don't go emotional with it though as that can lead to emotional reasoning, i.e. thinking errors).

At the end of the day, paying the price is just a choice. You must *choose to do it.* You must also continue to choose to do it on an ongoing basis. Yes, you will slip up and make bad choices, but that's okay, normal, and perfectly fine, just *choose to get back up and do better next time.*

TAKE ACTION

A healthy human has until the count of roughly two billion heartbeats before their eyes close forever. The count started at birth. It's counting now. Considering the macrocosm of time, this is such an ephemeral amount of time to be here that it's almost saddening. It would be a shame to cut this fleeting moment short because complications from the fat that we've accumulated ended up killing us. And it likely will kill us. Not directly, but obesity can lead to all those chronic metabolic diseases we keep hearing about (heart disease, cancer, stroke, diabetes—some of the leading causes of mortality).

However, fat is not always our fate (particularly if we don't surrender to it), and we don't lose it because we only ever think about losing it. We work at it. Every day until we achieve it. One kilogram at a time. Methodically, and, unfortunately, sometimes slowly. And there is one person that you can really trust on in all this, and that is *you.* It's you who must do it. You who must read the labels to find out what you're eating, who must cut out the abundant free sugars from what you're sticking in your mouth, who must give up the regular fruit juice, the fizzy drinks, the desserts. And you need to be confident in yourself and your ability to fix this problem, and you should be confident, for you are stardust!

I ask you, are you inspired? Or are you desperate? If we have neither then we generally end up doing nothing, and then 10 years pass and nothing has changed and we're still where we promised ourselves at one time we wouldn't be. It doesn't matter whether you're inspired or desperate, but whichever one it is, use it as the catalyst to start. To take action. And to start taking that action today. Procrastination is the thief of time, so give it no quarter, as every day we're getting older, and as we get older it becomes more and more difficult to win this battle, so don't let another day go by without changing course.

If you're still sitting there mulling it over thinking you'll start tomorrow, or planning to start tomorrow, or planning to plan to start tomorrow, you've already failed, because man plans and God laughs. So don't make plans, just make it happen.

Good luck.

PS. Cut down added sugar and fat and eat more plants.

Appendix 1
Q&A
(Common Questions & Queries)

I don't have time to cook. I've got work and kids and my life is manic!

It's certainly the case that eating well can take longer. But it's also certainly the case that losing fat often requires eating well (or monitoring your calories). You'll either have to shift your time slots around so you can accommodate the better food, or start cooking your food in a way that saves time at meal time so you can be eating well without having to invest a lot of time into it.

For instance, I am someone that very much dislikes cooking and so I do what I can to minimise the pain of having to cook it (because not eating well isn't an option I consider). So what I do is try and cook everything for the week on Sunday, which basically means the meat and sweet potatoes. I use frozen veg and microwave it for my meals. Last night I had gammon and veg. Prep time was ~5 minutes. This is comparable to the time a ready meal takes but yet accompanied by a level of nutrition and satiation that's much higher. I would suggest you do something like this also if your time is tight and you're always being pushed. Play around with the microwave timing on the veg so you can make the texture and consistency to what you like.

If the idea of completely planning or prepping your meals in advance is unreasonable then take moderate steps like we did with our food in general, i.e. make a conscious effort to plan one meal per week. Then, when one planned meal has become the norm for you, will yourself to plan another.

Are you sure this isn't a diet? Protein and fibre sounds like a diet to me?

Well, it's not just protein and fibre. It's protein, fibre, starch and fat (being particular to remember the healthy fats). So I guess if that's a diet then it's a diet, a type of holistic diet maybe, and I could certainly get on board with the idea if by diet we mean one of the original meanings of the word, which was "way of life". This is what every diet should be after all, because, as you know, the only diet plan worth considering is that one that you can stick to.

You're telling me to eat a lot of meat. Meat is fattening and the increased cancer risk makes this totally irresponsible.

Specifically, I'm advising protein, but yes, if you're a meat eater then a large portion of this is likely to come from animal sources, particularly meat. If you are a meat eater you should try and focus mostly on white meats (chicken/fish) as opposed to red meats. Red meat should certainly be lean cuts, which refers to 10% fat by weight (or extra lean, 5% fat by weight), as this will reduce the fat in the meat and therefore reduce the calories (bearing in mind that it can still sometimes be pretty high calorie).

Remember that we're using this high protein (e.g. meat) intake for its fat loss benefits (satiation, high digestive cost, as well as shifting the ratio of weight loss more towards fat and away from lean body mass), so whilst we are likely eating more protein than we require daily, it's only temporary, and we can shrink the portion of protein back when we've achieved our chosen fat levels.

As for health issues, it's important to keep in mind that the health risks associated with high meat intake, often given to us by way of a percentage increase to our risk, are mostly *relative* risk, not absolute risk (the same as most risk percentages we hear about in the media). So whilst we might be told that a certain amount of red meat intake increases our risk of colon cancer by ~20% (which actually refers to processed red meat[1]), this is actually a 20% increase to our baseline risk. As such, if our lifetime risk of developing colon cancer is

---

[1] Or is it lack of fibre. Or something else. The fact is *we don't know*, nor will we, because no one is going to sign up to a 30 year study in a hermetically sealed chamber in order to prove causality (and even *that* finding wouldn't necessarily apply to you as an individual). Meat eaters are also often more likely to eat more fat and less fibre. They can even eat more processed meat, which is quite often indicative of a more unhealthy lifestyle in general, such as forgoing exercise, even smoking. Any one of these, or something else, could account for that increased risk. What might be more surprising is that it's *only* 1%.

5%, a 20% increase to this is therefore an additional 1%, bringing our lifetime total to 6%. That's not great news, but perspective is important. Not to mention red meat being one of the most micro-nutrient dense foods that we can eat.

I'm also not personally aware of any studies that show the problems with animal protein (increased endotoxins, increased intestinal permeability, inflammatory problems, etc.) having held both fibre and fat constant (and various other things, depending on the study; most nutrition studies are also observational, which can't even answer the question). If these and other confounding factors aren't kept constant then nothing is necessarily being said about animal protein and we're jumping to conclusions. If these studies do exist then please let me know as I'd be very interested in reading them.

You should certainly be a little careful about eating out (in general as well as with meat) because food outlets not only drizzle fat and sugary stuff over everything to make it more tasty but they can also have access to meat cuts that are higher in fat than we can get from the supermarket ourselves. It's also not unknown for restaurants to lace the meat cuts with even more fat than what they came with originally (by dosing it with butter and stabbing it with a cocktail fork so the butter can seep in during cooking), so as to improve the flavour even more so.

Also be careful with food nutritional labeling as it can often be quite opaque, such that the labeling will list the, for example, saturated fat contained within the meat (or whatever the food is) as a percentage of daily allowance, but it will actually list this percentage *per serving* and not per piece of meat contained within the packet (and certainly not for the totality of what's contained within the packet). For example, a serving may be classified as 50g, but each joint of meat within the packet may be 200g, so eating a single joint of meat from within this packet means you're getting four times the amount of saturated fat that you thought you were getting from only a cursory reading of the label. So yes, spend a little time learning how to read labels, such as what's being classified as a serving and how big are the actual portions being given?

All in all, if you are a meat eater then try and lean mainly towards chicken and fish, and certainly non-processed meat (less fatty the better from a calorie perspective), learn what the label is telling you, sensibly prepare it yourself (don't add sugar or fat) and I don't see anything that should bother us about it (but have decent fibre intake).

Lastly, the gamut of nutrition science is pretty immature, and it's extremely difficult to get, let alone give, concrete, fundamental, blanket advice. The only advice that is somewhat robust enough to be said like that with a high degree of confidence, with the caveat that it is still somewhat a generalisation due to individual variability, is that we should eat fruit, veg, oily fish, and some wholegrain.

You didn't really cover what I'm meant to drink?

Water, ideally (plain or sparkling). Our bodies love this stuff and hydration is important for us to function properly. Other than that, just watch the sugar and calories, and don't have that coke with dinner, no meal deals, etc (unless they're diet/zero calorie).

Further to this, water/hydration increases our resting energy expenditure, and our resting energy expenditure is where most of our energy is used. Water should be drank cold for maximum energy expenditure as then your body has to use energy to heat it to your body temperature (it should be warmer for more rapid hydration, e.g. room/body temperature). Drink 500ml or so of it first thing upon waking since you're already dehydrated, and remember to drink when you're thirsty so you don't become so again. Remember to drink before you eat.

Any way to make it easier and/or speed up the process?

First, drink that water, but you can also exercise to speed up the process, both cardio and resistance. The benefits to fat loss can be huge if you're new to training, are very obese, or both. Routinely building muscle and having decent lean tissue also enables you to have a notably higher resting energy expenditure.

As for making it easier this really just depends on you enjoying what you eat. Fat loss requires consistency and consistency requires that you enjoy it because if you don't like it you're not going to always do it. Consistency also requires simplicity because then even when the going gets really tough and you're all out of discipline you can still implement it because it's a no-brainer—foods that you like plated up into percentages. Remember the food appendix, and anything there is valid for fat loss.

As for speed, a diet of raw food provides the fastest route to weight loss. Weight maintenance is even tricky to achieve on such a diet as the volume required is pretty extreme, but it can also be difficult to get a full compliment of nutrients on such a diet.

Don't take antibiotics unless absolutely necessary, as although this won't directly make it easier it will ensure that we don't make it any harder. We shouldn't be taking antibiotics willy-nilly anyway, but the less adversely affected our gut microbes are whilst we're losing fat the better.

I hear intermittent fasting, ketogenic, plant based diets, etc., are excellent at improving health markers like insulin resistance, diabetes, blood pressure, blood lipids, oxidative stress, and inflammation, so shouldn't I be on one of them?

It's true that these diets do improve these health markers, but any dieting method that results in fat loss will. The fact that all diets claim they improve the same health markers is revealing. It's all just marketing, such that instead of saying "losing fat improves numerous health markers" we can instead say that "plant based/keto/fasting improves numerous health markers". There will always be a new diet on the horizon claiming the same health benefits, the question though, is which one suits you?

You should also be extremely sceptical of grandiose claims. *Longevity* is a common one in the food and dieting world, but yet the only dietary choice that *seems like* it might show an increase to longevity is hunger by way of calorie restriction due to cleaning out the trash from our cells and compelling them to stay in survival mode (and too much of this is inferred from studies done on mice) —intense exercise and exposure to extremes of temperature do the same thing.

Is it true that high fat diets make me burn more fat and high carb diets make me store more fat? Doesn't this mean a high fat diet is best for losing fat?

Fat burning is not the same as fat loss. You do burn more fat on a high fat diet but that's only because you're eating more fat. You also store more fat on a high fat diet because, once again, you're eating more of it. Basically, on a high fat diet there's more fat being thrown around so you both burn and store more of it. However, what matters for overall fat balance is not whether you're eating carbs or fat or protein, but rather the calories over maintenance you're having of any of them. Remember, it's only *energy balance* that dictates how much fat you will store or burn, irrespective of where that calorie came from.

So a calorie is a calorie, and it only matters how many there are and not where they're coming from?

Whilst in the strictest of senses it's true that a calorie is a calorie, we don't want to view it like this because there's a danger it'll cause us to overlook the most important idea to keep in mind, and that's *nutrition.*

For example, I'm currently holding a *Cadbury's Double Decker* (yes, I eat these… and jelly sweets. Mmm), and the packet tells me it contains 250 calories (about 2/3rds from carbs and 1/3rd from fat). This is about 30 minutes on a treadmill at a pretty decent pace to burn off. Now compare that calorie count to, say, a tomato. If we take the tomato to have ~20 calories then we can eat 12 tomatoes for about the same calorie count. So yes, although we've eaten the same amount of calories whether we've had the Double Decker or the tomatoes, the nutritional value of the tomato is much higher; vitamin C, vitamin K, potassium, folate, and antioxidant lycopene (and no added sugar), all of which your body will thank you for. Moreover, the calories in the chocolate and fat are also much more readily available for absorption compared to the calories in a fibrous tomato, so whilst on paper the calories are the same in practice they will be very different.

We can actually make it even more explicit. I just went and bought a large dairy milk chocolate bar. It has 992 calories (let's call it an even 1000). My dinner last night consisted of sweet potatoes, couscous, chicken, mixed vegetables and a cheese sauce. It also had ~1000 calories. The difference here in nutritional value is huge (not to mention the calories available to us after the energy required to process and chew it will be considerably lower).

One more example. If a calorie was a calorie then 1 gram of fat could be considered the same as any other gram of fat, i.e. it would simply give us 9 calories of energy when absorbed. But we know this isn't so since mono-unsaturated and poly-unsaturated fats have a whole host of benefits that come with them, yet trans fat is nothing if not poison. Both are fat, and both provide the same energy when burned, but should we consider them synonymous?

Are you really telling me I don't have to count calories?

Although trying to lose fat means we're manipulating our calorie in-take in some way, this doesn't mean that we have to count the calories that we're eating, and I actually advise you not to. The reason for this is two-fold: First, it adds a workload to your nutrition, and an increased workload means that there's more for us to do and this can be irksome, get on our nerves, and make us quit. We don't want to be doing stuff like that if we don't want to. Second, you won't count calories accurately. You will always be off (and/or unknowingly under report your intake). It's sometimes argued that as long as you're consistently inaccurate with the calories then it's fine. This could be true, but unless you weigh all your food, calculate all the macros, and assume that all meat cuts have the same fat content then you don't know what calories you're eating anyway (nor can we realistically and reliably know how many calories we expend). The best we can ever do is achieve estimates in order to make a best guess.[2] There also looks to be a risk of developing disordered eating with calorie and macro counting as well as taking the joy out of it.

Alas, weigh and measure yourself instead (when you're leaner you can start looking in the mirror/taking photos). If you're losing weight (over the long term) then you're in a calorie deficit. If you're not then you're not so you need to eat less calories.

The point is that you don't need to count calories but you do need to eat *low calorie dense* and *satiating* food. This is fibre and protein (specifically the fibre and lean protein), so just increase protein and especially fibre to your maximum. If the protein is a meat source then be careful with the high calorie (i.e. fatty) meat (e.g. ground beef, steak, etc). Drink before you eat. *Eat slowly* so as to tap into your hunger and satiety cues (aim to finish *last* out of everyone you eat with. If you don't eat with people then time your standard eating, then extend it. Aim to double it). And don't order seconds until 20 minutes have passed and you'll be fine (and be sure you're not still eating when you're being told that you're getting full). Another worthwhile tip would be to eat in the order of protein > fibre > starch (or cut the starch out of whatever meals you're comfortable doing it with).

You do of course need to remember the added sugar, so *snack responsibly*, and be careful with the sauces and condiments that you're putting on things as these can just skyrocket the calories back up despite having designed your plate with appropriate portions. Also remember that eating healthy (nuts, avo-

---

[2] For your daily calorie intake, taking your weight (in lbs) and multiplying by 12–15 (sedentary–active) is as good a ballpark method as any for finding your maintenance values. Weighing yourself is still the gold standard as to whether these values are correct or not.

cado, etc) is not the same as eating to lose weight—something that many people routinely get wrong, including those who should know better, by having too much high calorie dense food "because it's healthy". Excessive fat on your body is unhealthy, irrespective of where the calories came from.

That said, if you want to count calories then you should do so. You should also do it if you want to eat a lot of high calorie dense foods. Just remember that you're doing it because you want to. And if you do want to then my recommendation would be to take a look into the flexible dieting approach. My goal throughout has been to try and get you to self-regulate and see how you can intuit your foodstuffs, with the end goal of removing the need to count.

Fibre bloats and makes me feel weird and there be much activity down below! Help!

You raised your fibre intake too fast. Cut back until the symptoms fade and then progress forward again, but slower. How slow? *As slow as necessary.* If onions or beans make your gut irritable then add a shaving or a bean to a pound of other stuff, then add some more when it feels like your gut has learned what it's doing with them. The goal is diversity of plants (and food in general), so do the same for any other produce that you experience issues with (or just don't eat it).

You really can't rush your fibre uptake as your gut can't take it. Your gut is adaptable but you need to build up gradually, changing the ratio of the bacteria in your gut so they know how to deal with what you're feeding them in order for you to be able to gain all the benefits and nutrients possible from this stuff (look at it as training your gut over time). A low fibre intake up to now has made it so you won't have as many of the bacteria in your gut that deal with this stuff and so you'll end up overloading it. If you don't build up slowly then you also won't be as satiated as you can be and you'll just end up bloated and likely backed up.

If you're feeling particularly bloated or unsettled for a protracted period of time then eat a bit of rubbish. The rubbish can be whatever you used to eat, like chips and beans, some fast food burger (don't get the meal deal), a slice of pizza, etc. This will most likely sort you out, but don't rush your fibre uptake next time.

Be sure to also drink more water as your water consumption needs to go up if your fibre intake does.

I want to continue to eat lots of things with added sugar and not cut down on them yet still lose fat, how?

Well, if you want to eat lots of sugary things then you'll have to start counting your calories (or having a daily and consistent very high output). If you're eating lots of things with added sugar and/or fat then calories are going to rack up pretty fast and you're not going to be satiated from most of them, so you'll overshoot your maintenance levels by some margin if you don't quantify or burn them off like crazy. You are also more than likely going to be routinely hungry with the high sugar route. But sure, count your calories and of course you can lose fat on such a diet.

Counting calories allows us to just cut x number of calories to bring us into a calorie deficit (although calorie counting for weight loss targets isn't as straightforward as it sounds[3]), and for pure energy balance purposes all fuel sources are equivalent (that is, they are energy).

What about "cheat meals"?

My take on this is somewhat contrary to the rest of the health and fitness community, but by definition a cheat meal is when you *break your strict diet rules* and have something you shouldn't. It's commonly viewed as a type of saving grace at keeping you on track with your diet choices. There are a number of arguments in favour of it, but the main, somewhat quantifiable sounding one, concerns *leptin*. The argument goes like this: Leptin is a hormone that is produced by fat cells. It does many things, including regulating fat storage, energy, and how many calories you eat and burn. Leptin levels go up when you eat, and when you have high enough levels in your system it tells your brain you've got enough fat and don't need to eat more. When levels drop it sends signals to your brain that you need to eat. Basically, leptin goes up when you eat which tells you to stop, and it goes down when fat declines telling you to start. It's like a type of negative feedback loop that's continuously cycling around your system telling you to start eating and to stop eating. As such, eating a cheat meal (gen-

---

[3] E.g. Let's say you're 100kg and want to lose 1% per week. One percent of 100kg is 1kg, and 1kg of fat is 7800 calories, which would give us our daily calorie deficit as $7800 / 7 = 1115$ (whether through input, output, or both). Next week you're 99kg, etc. As you can see, calorie deficit will decrease linearly with our weight, so when we've got down to, say, 70kg, 1% of this will be 700g, which would give us our daily calorie deficit as $(7800 \times 0.7) / 7 = 780$.

erally high calorie, fat and sugar) sends leptin through the roof, tricking the hormone cycle into producing more leptin temporarily and therefore suppressing your desire to overeat too often. Thus, having a cheat meal every now and then is a good idea because it'll satiate your body's desire to eat rubbish by piling on the fat. Additional fat means leptin levels will stay high for a while so you can eat healthy for longer and continue to be happy about it.

Now, I'm no endocrinologist or biochemist, but this argument seems a little strange to me, for when, in our evolution, would leptin have been required to send signals to the brain telling us that we have enough fat? Well, never. So why would something that wasn't used or needed have given such an adaptive benefit to the carriers that it spread like wildfire through the gene pool? It wouldn't have.

Our bodies function the complete opposite to this in fact and our evolution has designed us to keep eating. Consider the dessert tummy effect: we've just munched our way through an over-sized 3-course meal and we're stuffed. Feeling wrong and maybe a little ill... don't touch the belly! But yet they bring out the dessert menu and that chocolate gateau starts to look rather appealing. Maybe we can squeeze in a little more after all. The brain starts to value different quality calories when we're in this condition, calories that are crammed into as small a space as possible so they can be squeezed into every nook and cranny we have remaining. The more calorically dense the food the more the brain likes it, vis-à-vis, desserts.[4] The genes that code for this effect managed to make their way through the gene pool due to the advantage that developing a calorie buffer gave to our ancestors in their environment. This design is not negated because we've eaten a plate of chips, beans and sausage. Besides, if satiety was the result of leptin then we should be able to fix obesity with leptin injections, but it's been tried and was found wanting (much to the likely disappointment of Amgen). Further, digestive system hormones such as *glucagon-like peptide* (GLP-1) and *cholecystokinin* (CCK) are what increase after eating to increase satiety and reduce hunger, and they work independently of leptin levels and body fat. The obese also appear to have trouble with their leptin signaling so I'm not sure what use the leptin argument would have for them anyway.

---

[4] It's the same thing that, for example, bears do when they're getting full from gorging on fish and so no longer eat the entire fish but rather resort to eating only the fat and skin. Not much of a dessert to us, for sure, but it's the same mechanism.

From what I can make out, leptin would be the starvation hormone, not the satiety hormone. It's biological role is to turn on the starvation response (that which compels us to view our partner's thighs as appetising sometime after our plane has crashed in the Andes), not to stop us from eating (whether specifically sugar and fat or otherwise), since its function appears when we don't have enough of it, because when we don't have enough of it we don't have any fat, and, therefore, we're starving. Besides, we're not going to stop eating fat (or sugars). Fats are important and they should always be part of a healthy nutrition plan. There's also other arguments in favour of cheat meals, such as the ghrelin one and ones relating to thyroid hormones that come into play with sustained low-carb diets.

Either way, this line of reasoning and its implications don't actually concern us. For a start, we're not cutting entire chains of energy out of our life, and we're not on a 'diet' because they're just not reliable enough. Yes, there are success stories, but that's no indication of them being reliable for any particular individual. The idea of a cheat meal is because sticking to a new behaviour is hard before it's formed into an agreeable and likeable habit, so every now and then you're allowed to break the behaviour and go back to your old-self easing the pressure of your new, enforced, behaviour.

I actually believe there's a danger here with this idea of enforced new habits (which implies you don't like them) and with them being hard (which implies an assumed cold turkey approach). For example, let's say you've decided that your cheat meal or day is going to be on Saturday. So all week long you go cold turkey and punish yourself with your new eating habits, longing for Saturday to roll around so you can finally eat something tasty. That's like enforcing cold turkey on a heroin addict all week long and then giving them the needle for the weekend. That isn't what we do. We give them morphine and wean them. You're advised not to go cold turkey if you currently eat a lot of 'bad stuff', and the purpose of this is to take the pressure off and break into your new habits slowly without enforcing anything that will cause discomfort and anxiety. We're not concerned about you eating well for a month or two or six or a year. We're concerned about you eating well for the next 50 years. We changed slowly so as to set you up for this success.

Further, there's a hidden implication to the idea of cheat meal and that is that you're 'cheating yourself away' from that which you don't like doing. This just sounds like the beginning of a disaster and you shouldn't feel it necessary to cheat yourself away from anything. You're not disliking your food for every meal of the week apart from the one that you enjoy. You *must enjoy* what you eat. If you don't you'll just fail.

The sooner you identify the things you like and can live on the better. The added benefit to this is that your choices are going to stick around with you long term and not just throughout some half-cocked diet that you can only exist in for a small slice of your life before you're off it. And that's exactly what we're doing here: we're changing our lifestyle, *forever*.

To me, cheat meals make more sense as a psychological hack rather than a physiological one.[5] It helps those who don't really enjoy what they're eating and are somewhat forcing themselves to eat healthy foods but yet never truly get on-board with a healthy nutrition plan and lifestyle. The amount of times I've heard or read someone say something like *"I was going crazy until I had my cheat meal... but after having it I was perfectly content to get back to business. Cheat meals rule!"*, just adds weight to this line of reasoning. This way of proceeding is anything but optimal as you're constantly fighting it. There's no possible end to this merry-go-round either, so try not to get on.

Cheat meals are certainly unnecessary (although not a disaster, and better viewed as a *treat* meal), and a low body fat percentage and a decent amount of lean tissue actually enables you to eat a lot of the crap you want to anyway (although still in moderation, assuming your goal isn't to be shredded) since the lean tissue is a product of working out so you have a higher energy expenditure (including resting) and have bigger glycogen stores, but you need to get down there first.

However, if a cheat meal or diet break takes the pressure off you psychologically every once in a while then feel free to partake in it. Eating rubbish for one or two meals a week, or dieting for 2–6 weeks then going back to maintenance for a week, so as to keep yourself sane is better than the alternative of eating lots of rubbish all the time. But don't go crazy; *be mindful*.

---

[5] Although some people do show an increase to their metabolic rate in the short-term. This still doesn't equate to greater fat loss, however.

Can I target fat loss? I like my bum but I want to thin out my face.

You may have seen various magazine and internet articles, guides and even books on your travels about how you can do this sort of stuff, such as lose belly fat, face fat, butt fat, thigh fat, etc. This seems to be done solely for marketing and SEO (Search Engine Optimisation) purposes, since it's known that people look and search for information on this stuff, so guides and articles are written on it so as to capture the attention of the people looking for it in order to sell them something (or serve up adverts and additional marketing to them).

In truth, you can only lose fat, and you have no control over where your personal fat gets lost first. Generally speaking, you'll lose your fat stores first in the areas where you have the most stored (such as men losing it around the waist and women losing it below the waist) simply because there is more fat in those areas that can be tapped into for fuel. There are also places where fat is particularly troublesome to remove (like lower-back fat), but this is just how it works and no amount of fancy eating plans or patterns will change this.

Exercising the muscles in areas can lead to more tone, of course, but if there's too much fat it's not going to make much of a difference to the way the area looks because there's fat covering up the muscle. After all, toned looking abs are built in the kitchen, not the gym, since the first step is losing the covering fat, not ab exercises.

What to do about hunger?

First, realise there's nothing wrong with an empty stomach, and a rumbling stomach is not a cue that you need to eat but is actually your system cleaning up the last remaining remnants of what you had previously. Feelings of hunger also don't climb linearly (nor exponentially!). They come in waves, so push through and the pang will reduce. Hunger is also a sensation that you can get used to and feel comfortable with over time. Lastly, if you're underfeeding then hunger is going to be a thing sometimes.

Here are 8 things that can help:

1. Stay hydrated. Although not dealing with hunger directly it's included here for three reasons: first is that being hydrated just makes you feel all round better. Second is that thirst can be mistaken for hunger, so staying hydrated ensures this doesn't apply and you won't feel hungry and eat additional calories when really you're thirsty. And third, water also fills you up. It should be plain or sparkling water as there is no substitute for water. Drop a slice of fruit or veg in it if you require a different taste.

2. Drink coffee or tea (with caffeine). Can work well for appetite control on some people. It's also a stimulant, which causes you to burn more energy.

3. Eat vegetable soup. You can eat this before your meals, too, since you'll likely end up eating fewer calories with your actual meal.

4. Have dairy or a few teaspoons of Greek yogurt. The reason this works is that these foods contain *whey* and/or *casein,* which are decent for satiation. The dryer the cheese the less lactose.

5. Homemade Protein Milkshake or Ice Cream. Good amount of bulk, lots of protein, and tasty!

6. Non-Calorie Dense Foods. You can load up on these. Eat the biggest salad you've ever seen (for example). Make it tasty with low-calorie condiments—don't add 500 calories to it with sauces. Also do this type of thing before you binge, and add a big glass of water as well.

7. Hard Cardio. If you push hard with your cardio workouts (such as running/cycling hard for 30–60 minutes) it will ruin your appetite and make you not want to eat.

8. Sleep. Remember to get enough sleep. We don't want ghrelin the gremlin putting a spanner in the works.

Genes or Environment?

Our genes make us human, and being human means we're a readily fattening, sugar and fat seeking, inherently lazy species that's been put into a cheap, super abundant sugar and fat environment that allows easy acquisition of both. As such, I don't think an either/or question has much value.

It's also not just a case of our food environment changing but nearly everything about our environment has changed from the environments that we evolved to thrive in (physical exertion and calorie shortages). Consider a modern work environment of affluent nations and we can see that many do little in the way of physical exertion. For instance, sitting at this computer typing these words costs me about 100 calories an hour. Compare this to, say, a coal miner, who would be burning over 400 calories an hour. That's a 12,000 calorie difference over the course of a 5 day week. In a full year I will have expended 624,000 fewer calories, enough energy for me to run over 270 marathons. Lest you think I've stacked the deck by choosing a non-physically demanding profession and pitting it against a physically demanding one, consider the difference between an electric sewing machine (~70 cal/hr) and an old foot-driven sewing machine (~100 cal/hr). Well the answer here is just 1 power of 10 less than previous, so 62,400 calories a year, which is enough energy for me to run 27 marathons.

As for what the real reason is that we have an obesity problem, I don't think we can point to anything in particular and say that's the singular, ultimate cause (save for more calories in than out because there's no denying that). Things are seldom either/or. Rather it's a combination of everything acting in concert (genes, food, culture).

Since we cannot yet effectively change our genes to help us out, nor does an individual have much influence on culture over the course of their lifetime, we're left with having to deal with our food environment. This is no bad thing because our culture is marvellous and our genes haven't changed from what they were previous. That is, they still design us to be hunting and gathering endurance athletes.

I don't wish to downplay the power of genes (and I initially planned a chapter dedicated to genes or the environment but felt it detracted from the book's focus) as our genes certainly *predispose* us to a whole host of conditions and behaviours, but we are what we eat (and do and are exposed to). Genes do not place us in a small box. Rather genes enclose us in a bracket encompassing a wide range of potential. So whilst we might not be able to achieve the exact form of our favourite celebrity this doesn't mean that we can't get better if we make the choices that align to doing so.

What about the gut microbiome? When this goes awry it causes obesity, no?

It could be a proximate cause and a predisposition, but *calories* cause obesity. As such, the causal arrow can't even be close to clear. What is clear though is that the obese and lean have different ratios of the various gut bacteria, and it looks like we can shift the obese folks ratios into the ratios of the lean folks: We can take *probiotics* in an attempt to help repopulate our gut with beneficial bacteria, but probiotics, like diets, mostly only work whilst we're on them (and that's assuming the microbes we have already actually allow the probiotic ones to graft on since it's somewhat a case of first come first served). When we stop taking them the benefits also often stop. Taking probiotics but continuing to eat a lot of rubbish isn't going to do much to help our bacteria over the longer term because we're not actually fixing anything with our diet to aid their population. So *prebiotics* is what we can take to enhance and replenish the very healthiest strains of our gut bacteria, and fibre is a prebiotic. Little surprise that we again come back to fibre. Fibre actually provides so many benefits (including reducing appetite, increasing insulin sensitivity, and encouraging weight loss directly) that the case is all but closed in respect to its efficacy in aiding fat loss (and health in general). Just eat more of it (and the more diversity the better) and let your gut microbes do the rest... but don't forget to increase your intake of it gradually.

What about antibiotics? After all, they make livestock fat and the time frame fits with our obesity problem?

Somewhat the same question as the previous one really but yes, it's interesting. Obesity is a complicated problem. There are no-doubt a number of contributing factors, even innocent things like being born by Cesarean section or brought up on formula can uptick our risk percentage of obesity, so it would be no surprise if something which kills bacteria, of which we have a symbiotic relationship several trillion strong, also affected us in profound ways (especially considering their role in our digestion and immune responses). Indeed, it's not just obesity that's complicated but *everything* about reality is complicated.

However, antibiotics save lives so we should continue to take them (when absolutely necessary that is; they do nothing for a cold or the flu or any virus), not to mention we can do nothing about whether we were born through the gates to the world or lifted out through the stomach, breast fed or brought up on formula (neither combination of which leads necessarily to obesity), but we can do something about our food. And *we can fix* the problem with our food.

Women?

Women and men are different (despite what the internet seems to determined in trying to convince us of), so approaching fat loss with the sexes one-to-one is not the best of ideas. For example, women are more efficient with energy than men are, and so they gain fat easier and hold onto it better, which is, once again, just an evolutionary fitness adaption that helps you have the energy available for your offspring. Premenopausal women are also generally more prone to accumulating subcutaneous fat, which is less sensitive to the signals that break the fat apart for burning and more sensitive to the signals that promote its storage, therefore making the fat that you likely want to lose (back of the arms, hips, butt, thighs) more resistant to being shifted (this can often change post menopause where you can become more susceptible to visceral fat storage).[6]

The menstrual cycle further complicates the issue due to the changing hormones being thrown around all over the place, such as changing oestrogen levels causing a change in serotonin levels, which throws your mood out of whack; a low mood can compel us to seek something to alleviate it, such as dopamine. Since food can cause a dopamine release, food can therefore be a route to increased pleasure and elevated mood.

However, fat is still fat, and fat loss is just fat loss, so a calorie deficit does mean you lose it (it's just that, as a woman, it will likely take you longer). You should certainly learn your menstrual cycle and not fight your physiology, such that if you feel terrible then maybe go easier on yourself; if you don't then don't. Here are some pointers:

- Changes in your body week to week are likely to cause more fluctuations in bodyweight but this shouldn't be construed as you falling off the wagon (e.g. water retention alone can add up to a few percent of body weight). You should judge yourself week to week because of this instead, such that the weighing yourself daily and taking the average over the week that I gave you in the chapter on how to not fail should be done in weekly isolation rather than as a continuous thing. For instance, don't compare your weight in the 2 weeks leading up to ovulation to the 2 weeks following it. Separate the weeks and focus on them one at a time.

---

[6] Of course, these are generalisations; not all women carry their fat in these areas, just like not all men carry their fat in the belly.

- You will seem to gain fat easier in the two weeks following ovulation than in the two weeks leading up to it because you're burning more calories (quite likely the result of hormone-driven temperature changes), which compels you to binge on something to offset the cravings you're having because of it. The trouble here is you overshoot, consuming ~500 extra calories when you're only burning ~200 extra calories. Try and offset these cravings after ovulation by indulging in something healthy (e.g. an extra couple of pieces of fruit a day). Certainly don't binge on anything inappropriate.

- Don't start on a diet after ovulation as you're just making it harder on yourself. Instead, start on a diet at the beginning of the 2 weeks leading up to ovulation to give yourself an easier time.

- Start lifting Weights (this applies to men, too). Generally speaking, the older we get the less lean tissue we still have on our frame as we lose it quite rapidly if we don't maintain it, especially in our later years (and we lose it even faster if we're in a calorie deficit). As such, lifting weights will bring back and develop our lean tissue. This burns energy with the activity, additional energy from the muscle (which assists in losing the weight initially and keeping it off long term), increases available glycogen stores (1–2% of muscle mass), improves glucose tolerance, and will make you feel good. Muscle is so good for us for so many reasons that everyone should be doing resistance training. Everyone. Train hard, but remember to go easy at first.

- Hit the gym when your testosterone is spiking just before ovulation (when you start to feel hornier than normal) and you can ratchet up your calorie burn considerably. After ovulation, oestrogen and progesterone levels are up, promoting fat burning.

- Lastly, remember that you have a higher body fat percentage for a reason, so don't go crazy thinking that the mid to low teens is a good idea. Such a low body fat percentage on a woman is almost certainly unhealthy (single digits is fatal). The most shredded bikini model you're ever likely to see will be 15% (most will be higher) and she'll be feeling like absolute crap due to having so little energy.

Appendix 2

How To Read
Nutrition Labels

Although touched on previously, I thought it best to make it explicit here so you know what you're looking at. I mainly have condiment labels in mind when writing this because an abundance of calories (several hundred) can easily fly under the radar throughout the day with this stuff, but everything said here can be transferred to any label you encounter.

This section also isn't meant to imply that you should be reading all labels all the time, but rather to give you the information necessary to ensure that your condiments aren't ruining your fat loss efforts; having the majority of your food as low calorie dense is for nothing if we're just skyrocketing the calories back up with our condiments.

It's also worth knowing that the calories (and macronutrients) given on nutritional labels are not always accurate. This can be due to a rounding of the calorie numbers and/or the weight of the object (e.g. spraying oil listed as 0 calories when really it's 9 calories per gram (it's fat), or a wrap listed as 100g when really it's 115g).

It's not that the labels are wilfully misleading us, it's just that they're allowed to round off calorie numbers and/or take averages (plus it's not always possible to be exact, due, in part, to foods being biological and therefore exhibit variation).

Either way, the result is the same on our end; incorrect calorie amounts. And to not be at the complete mercy of this misinformation it can help to remember the following:

Protein = 4 calories per gram

Carbs = 4 calories per gram

Fat = 9 calories per gram.

Fibre is often not found on nutrition labels because the majority of the time it's been stripped out, but if you do find it on one then you can either calculate it as 4 calories per gram like the other carbohydrates or as 2.5 calories per gram (which is the average of 2–3 calories).

That's all you need to remember. And with that, here is an example label from a condiment:

Servings per bottle -30		
Typical values	Per 100g	Per serving (15g)
Energy	435kJ	65kJ
	102kcal	15kcal
Fat	0.1g	Trace
-of which saturates	Trace	Trace
Carbohydrate	23.2g	3.5g
-of which sugars	22.8g	3.4g
Protein	1.2g	0.2g
Salt	1.8g	0.3g

First up is *servings*, and although this label has a per serving column on the right at 15g, this isn't always the case as many will just list the serving without an actual value next to it (serving size will be found elsewhere on the label), leaving us with having to work out the servings ourselves from the other values. In such a case we could look at the top of the above label where it tells us that it contains 30 servings, and given that the contents of the bottle is 460g, a serving would be 460 / 30 = 15.3g.

For condiments this is a common case since 15g is often comparable to 15ml, which is a tablespoon's worth. Generally, the more viscous the condiment the more chance there is of the listing being in weight rather than in volume. But either way, we should first pay attention to the serving so we're on the same page with what the label is telling us.

This label also tells us that a serving is said to have 15kcal, which is just 15 calories to you and I because that's how we talk about calories in everyday parlance even though it's not strictly accurate. The 65kJ listing is because joule, like calorie, is just a name for a unit of energy.

Anyway, to work out the energy value for what we're having we need to look at the *macronutrients* (protein, carbs and fat). This label tell us that there's 0.2g of protein, 3.5g of carbs, and a trace of fat (that we can comfortably ignore). This gives us an energy value per serving (15g) of 4 x 0.2 (for the protein) + 4 x 3.5 (for the carbs) = 14.8 calories per serving, which the label rounded up and so can be considered spot on... well done *Heinz!*

This isn't always the case with labels. For example, a loaf of bread I have in the cupboard lists the slices as 42g with 93 calories each, but I've just weighed every slice and the average slice weight for the loaf was 45g. That's ~7% more weight, so we can assume it's 7% more of each macronutrient, which for the sake of this example we'll assume gives us 7% more calories. So rather than the listed 93 calories per slice we're at ~100 calories per slice. That's not necessarily make or break with this example, but it's worth knowing.

Of course, I'm certainly not recommending that you weigh or measure out your condiment servings, but knowing how many calories there are to a tablespoon is knowledge that you can use to make informed decisions about how much of what you're putting on things. And that's important because condiments alone have the ability to prevent your fat from being lost, irrespective of how well you're doing with everything else.

Go and take a look at a nutrition label with this knowledge in mind to prove to yourself that you understand what you've just read.

Lastly, before we leave this section, let's understand alcohol. The weight of alcohol is 0.8g per ml and it's 7 calories per gram. So if we have an alcoholi drink that is 40% alcohol that means it's 40% by volume (ml). If we drink 500m of such a drink then we've drunk 500 x 0.4 = 200ml of alcohol. To find the weigh of the alcohol we multiply the volume by 0.8. This would give us 200 x 0.8 = 160 of alcohol. We then multiply the weight of the alcohol by the calories (160 x 7) an we've got a total of 1120 calories in this example.

Alcoholic drinks can also have sugar, sometimes quite a bit such as in variou wines and liqueurs, but, in general, most of the calories will come by way of th alcohol, not the added sugar.

If it helps and makes it easier, you can just work out alcoholic calories b assuming that 1ml = 1g as this will remove a step in the calculation. The result o doing this just means that your calorie calculation is 20% higher than it actually is

Appendix 3

Sugar Names

An ingredients list can often contain more than one sugar, sometimes multiple. It won't list the quantity (and they're not going to since the quantities of ingredients are guarded secrets for obvious reasons), but the position of the ingredient in the list indicates the relation of that ingredient to the other ingredients. Sometimes a percentage will be given for another ingredient, so you can know if it 'has more than this' or 'less than this'. This is far from perfect, but sometimes it can give you a worthy tell. Either way, as you know, avoid as much added sugar as you're comfortable with whilst pursuing fat loss.

To remind you, *sucrose* is table sugar, which is 50/50 glucose/fructose. Glucose is the energy. Fructose is the sweetness.

The following list is relatively extensive for ingredients, but not exhaustive. Most things ending in -*ose* are sugars.

> **Agave Nectar** - 70–90% fructose
>
> **Barley malt** - Various sugars (incl. glucose, maltose)
>
> **Beet sugar** - Sucrose that hasn't been processed with bone char, making it acceptable to vegans and vegetarians
>
> **Blackstrap molasses / Treacle** - Refined cane/beets sugar (sucrose amount varies)

Brown rice syrup - Glucose

Brown sugar - Sucrose with added molasses

Buttered syrup - Syrup made from butter

Cane Juice Crystals - Liquid extracted from sugar cane (sucrose)

Cane Sugar - Sucrose

Caramel - A variety of sugars (will contain fructose)

Carbohydrate - Most often, in nutrition, used to identify a group commonly referred to as sugars

Carob syrup - Will contain fructose

Caster sugar - Sucrose

Coconut sugar - 70–80% sucrose

Confectioner's sugar - Sucrose

Corn syrup - Glucose

Corn syrup solids - Dehydrated corn syrup (glucose)

Date sugar - 60% sucrose

Demerara sugar - Sucrose with added molasses (~90% sucrose)

Dextrin - Glucose (broken down starch)

Dextrose - Chemically identical to glucose. Made from corn

Diastatic malt - Contains sucrose and fructose

Evaporated cane juice - Consider it sucrose

Florida crystals - Consider it sucrose

Fructose - Fruit sugar. Has the sweetest taste

Galactose - Very similar to glucose

Glucose - The body's first source of fuel

Glucose-Fructose - UK/EU naming of High-Fructose corn syrup (HFCS)

Glucose solids - Glucose

Golden sugar - Sucrose with some molasses

Golden syrup - Sucrose

Grape sugar - Glucose

High-Fructose corn syrup (HFCS) - Often appended with a number indicating fructose percentage, e.g. HFCS 42/55/90

Honey - Sucrose (fibre, protein and fat amount varies)

Icing sugar - Sucrose

Isomaltose - Glucose/glucose

Isomalutose - Glucose/fructose (absorbed slower than sucrose, potentially beneficial to diabetics)

Invert sugar - Sucrose

Lactose - Milk sugar (glucose and galactose)

Malt syrup - ~65% maltose (glucose), ~30% carbohydrate, ~3% protein

Maltitol - Nearly identical to sucrose but less sweet (sugar alcohol)

Maltodextrin - Similar to corn syrup solids (glucose) but with less sugar

Maltose - Glucose/glucose. The stuff that's in beer.

Mannose (D-Mannose) - Glucose

Maple syrup - High in sucrose

Molasses / Treacle - Refined cane/beets sugar (sucrose amount varies)

Muscovado sugar - Sucrose

Panela sugar - Sucrose

Raw sugar - Sucrose with some molasses

Refiner's syrup - Golden syrup (sucrose)

Rice syrup - Glucose

Sorghum syrup - ~45% sucrose, ~15% glucose, ~15% fructose, plus water

Sucanat - Unrefined cane sugar (sucrose)

Sucrose - Cane or beet sugar. 50/50 Glucose/Fructose

Tagatose (D-Tagatose) - Like fructose but made from cow's milk (whey)

Treacle sugar - Sucrose

Trehalose - Glucose/glucose.

Trehalulose - Glucose/fructose

Turbinado sugar - Sucrose with some molasses

Yellow sugar - Brown sugar (sucrose)

Appendix 4
Fruit

This might seem like a strange thing to include as fruit is good for us, right? Indeed it is, but many modern fruits have been engineered to be much sweeter than their wild ancestors and so are more calorie dense. Of course, eating fruit is still not like drinking liquid sugar as the sugar is wrapped up in the fibre (eating fruit can be a wise choice if you have a sweet tooth), but if you're at a high-body fat percentage (40%+) and want to be more strict with your calorie intake then you may want to try and stay away from the fruits with the high calories and sugar content anyway as this just limits your calorie intake even more.

The following figures are calories, sugar and fibre per ~100g of fruit. They are not exact. Eat fresh or frozen, and try to avoid blending or juicing fruit when in pursuit of fat loss as it just turns it into liquid sugar. Careful with dried stuff (and better to just avoid it).

Apple - 52 cal / 10g sugar / 2.4g fibre

Apricot - 48 cal / 9g sugar / 2g fibre

Avocado - 161 cal / 0.7g sugar / 6.5g fibre

Banana - 105 cal / 14g sugar / 3.1g fibre

Blackberries - 42 cal / 4.8g sugar / 5.1g fibre

Blueberries - 55 cal / 10g sugar / 2.1g fibre

Cherimoya - 76 cal / 13g sugar / 3.1g fibre

Cherries (sour) - 50 cal / 8.5g / 1.6g fibre

Cherries (sweet) - 63 cal / 13g sugar / 2.1g fibre

Clementine - 47 cal / 9.3g / 1.8g fibre

Dates - 280 cal / 63g sugar / 8g fibre

Fig - 74 cal / 16g sugar / 3g fibre

Grapefruit - 42 cal / 6.8g sugar / 1.6g fibre

Grapes - 70 cal / 15.2g sugar / 0.9g fibre (also moreish!)

Guava - 67 cal / 9g sugar / 5.3g fibre

Jackfruit - 94 cal / 18.6g sugar / 1.5g fibre

Kiwi - 61 cal / 9g sugar / 3g fibre

Lemon - 29 cal / 2.5g sugar / 2.9g fibre

Lime - 30 cal / 1.6g sugar / 2.8g fibre

Mango - 61 cal / 14g sugar / 1.6g fibre

Melon - 34 cal / 8g sugar / 1g fibre

Nectarine - 45 cal / 7.8g sugar / 1.8g fibre

Orange - 50 cal / 8.4 sugar / 2.2g fibre

Papaya - 43 cal / 7.7g sugar / 1.8g fibre

Passion Fruit - 97 cal / 11g sugar / 10.5g fibre

Peach - 40 cal / 9g sugar / 1.6g fibre

Pear - 57 cal / 9.6g sugar / 3.1g fibre

Persimmons - 71 cal / 12.6g sugar / 3.6g fibre

Pineapple - 50 cal / 9.7g sugar / 1.4g fibre

Plum - 45 cal / 9.8g sugar / 1.4g fibre

Pomegranate - 83 cal / 13.6g sugar / 3.8g fibre

Raisins - 303 cal / 59g sugar / 3.8g fibre

Raspberries - 50 cal / 4.5g sugar / 6.5g fibre

Strawberries - 32 cal / 4.8g sugar / 2g fibre

Tangerine - 53 cal / 10.2g sugar / 1.8g fibre

Tomato - 18 cal / 2.6g sugar / 1.2g fibre

Watermelon - 30 cal / 6.3g sugar / 0.4g fibre

Appendix 5

How To Eat Healthy When Money Is Tight

The two fixes that I gave you (restrict added sugar and focus on the satiating foods of protein and fibre) are key, and I make it sound so simple, and for a lot of people it is, yet for another lot of people this might not be such a simple exercise. Poor areas are sparse with supermarkets and rammed with convenience stores that sell mostly processed food (which is crammed with sugar and fat) since it's cheaper and has a greater shelf-life, leading to these two things being not so easy after all.

Of course, higher energy dense food makes it so the energy cost goes down, which, on the face of it, seems like a good thing (more calories for less buck), but it's not a good thing when you're over consuming (which you are if you're overweight). As such, you can afford to get less calories because the reduction in calories will result in a reduction to your fat, which will result in an increase to your health.

However, that makes it sound so simple when really there's no simple answer to this problem. On the one hand, if you want to lose your fat then you really ought to do these two things. On the other hand, doing these two things can be difficult since not only are you fighting your wallet but you're also fighting the food availability. The internet opens up opportunity if you can get some access time as many things can be bought conveniently and for less money.

One of my first thoughts is that you're going to want a freezer (try the scrap yard. Many of these will still work, they've just been thrown away as it's easier than giving it away or selling it) and buy frozen stuff, in bulk, when things are in their season (plus this will save you money not having to commute so often). It's just as good as fresh (and can actually be better since it's frozen at source and never defrosted, disallowing degradation), and it's often cheaper. Chicken can be a cheap meat if you have a way to cook it. Buy it, cook it, cut it into daily portions and freeze it. Take one out a day. Forget steaming and roasting veg, just microwave it.

Here is some brainstorming that could help:

Don't have dependencies: Children, pets, dependent partners. Each of these costs a fortune.

Buy in bulk and in season: Things are often cheaper in bulk and also cheaper in season.

Don't impulse buy: The cost of impulse purchases racks up pretty fast. Stick to your list.

Don't throw food away: Stick it back in the fridge or freezer.

Consider home delivery: I pay £1 for home delivery. It'd cost me plenty more than that to drive. The added benefit to this is that you aren't browsing enticing sugary stuff. Even if you diligently shop on the periphery of a store it's not as selective as a specific search (plus there's plenty of things worth avoiding in the periphery sections and things you don't need to avoid in the middle).

Join a food co-op or SHARE program: Both viable ways to save money on food.

Buy groceries and protein when on sale: Even if you don't currently need it, because you will do.

Shop early morning or late: Stores often put reduced stuff out in the morning or it goes on sale in the evening. Buy these and, if necessary, freeze them (as long as you freeze on or before their use-by date then it's still in date).

Eat spinach: Spinach is nutritious bulk, and it's often cheap.

Eat kale: Kale is also nutritious bulk, and it's also often cheap.

Eat carrots, cabbage and onions: These are healthy, often cheap, and the carrots and cabbage will fill you up.

Consider moving to a rural area: Yes, there are more opportunities in urban areas but cost of living is often a lot higher.

Monitor prices: Make a note of the prices of your regular things so you know when they're up and when they're down.

Balance the books: Make a note of everything you and your family spend money on. Cut out the things that you can do without. Purchased computer software that came bundled with the computer when you bought it often catches people out. You likely don't need it.

Don't buy fancy brands: Generic stuff is a lot cheaper.

Give up smoking, drinking and drugs: They cost a fortune, even when done at a moderate level.

Appendix 6

Insulin Sensitivity

A contributing factor to not being satiated is you being insulin resistant. To fix this we need to become more insulin sensitive, and the main driver of insulin sensitivity is fat loss. However, we can also give it a helping hand as we go by employing various things, and we should do so since the whole body functions better when it's insulin sensitive (ignore that if you're a type-1 diabetic as it can sometimes increase the risk of hypoglycemia).

You can start the recovery process off by cutting down the foods that result in a strong insulin response (simple and refined carbs). If you want to continue to eat refined starches then try and make them resistant starches instead (unless you need the quicker energy for some reason and/or easier digestibility). Starch can be turned into a resistance starch by cooking it and then allowing it to cool. Whether you eat it cold or reheat it doesn't matter, it's still a resistant starch. Developing our lean tissue is also notable for increasing insulin sensitivity and improving our glucose tolerance.

Include whatever is agreeable to you from the following list to help increase insulin sensitivity even further. They're not magic bullets, so they won't be fixing your fat as if by a miracle. They're just little, additional helpers. And they will only help over time so consistency is key.

- Better sleep schedule
- Cinnamon (1tsp added to anything that's agreeable. Ceylon, not cassia)
- Eliminate added sugar
- Eliminate refined carbs (swap to wholegrain for everything)
- Exercise (both cardio and resistance)
- Fibre (eat lots. Be sure it has the soluble and the insoluble components still intact—don't blend it)
- Ginger (2–3g a day)
- Green tea
- Magnesium
- Mono & Poly Fats
- Reduce stress (train, meditate)
- Sleep (sleep deprivation causes insulin resistance)
- Vinegar (with the meal)

Appendix 7
Food

There might actually be a danger that you'll feel inundated or over-whelmed with the amount of items listed here, causing you not to take the time necessary to go through it and find what works for you. Try not to feel this way. You do not have to include everything. You also don't have to do it right now. Take your time. Do it at your leisure. My intention was to list as much as I thought necessary to not leave you wanting, not to overwhelm you.

My advice would be to quickly scan through each list and note some items that pique your interest and start with them, then come back every now and then when looking for some variety, an additional ingredient, or more information.

Try and get somewhat into recipe building. This is more important the more difficult your palate is to please—reaching for that dessert is not the an-swer you should be looking for, a more pleasing recipe is.

These lists obviously aren't exhaustive (far from it), but they can act as your starting point, and anything here can be plated up like we've discussed. You don't actually have to use this appendix for your food as long as you re-member the less than obvious stuff, like chicken being chicken and not chicken nuggets, and porridge is not a dessert, etc. Also notice that not all vegetables are created equal—parsnips, peas, sweetcorn, etc., are in the starch column, not fibre, and you can easily go into high calorie counts with this stuff.

For want of a better term, we're looking to eat 'real' foodstuffs, not foodstuffs that have had a lot of engineering gone into them. If you prefer to wander off on your own then you should check the labels. *Be mindful of your fat intake* and remember that there are 9 calories per gram of fat, 4 calories per gram of starch and protein, 2.5 calories per gram of fibre (as an average), and 7 calories per gram of alcohol (the body also preferentially metabolises alcohol for energy rather than fat). And remember to be mindful of your condiments, too.

Also, if you go on a largely strict fibre (carb) diet, such as plant based, vegetarian, vegan, etc., then be sure you get a full compliment of amino acids and you supplement for B12.

Lastly, the lower your body fat percentage becomes the more strict you have to be with your diet if you want to continue to progress.

MAIN INGREDIENTS

PROTEIN:	FIBRE (cals/100g):	STARCH (cals/100g):	SNACKS:
Cook meat separately so you can drain the fat and not have it absorb into the rest of the food.	Any fruit or veg. Use herbs and spices for flavour. Blanching, boiling, braising, roasting, sautéing. Boiling is generally the least healthy way to cook vegetables (unless it's a carrot).	Keep an eye out for lower calorie, lower carb, higher protein, higher fibre substitutes on pasta, bread and rice, e.g. *Ciaocarb, Exekiel, Flatout, ICON, Nupasta, Pedon, P28, Tumaro*, etc.	The best snacks are protein, but before you snack, *drink* (water, plain or sparkling, but anything calorie free). Get a little bowl or plate for your snacks—eat out the bag and you'll eat more.
- *Beef* - braised, casserole, grilled/broiled, ground, meatballs, pot-roast, roast chilli, steak (care with the fat, e.g. steak)	- *Apples* (52)	- *Acorn Squash* (57)	Care with low fat stuff as studies show that people eat considerably more of them, negating the benefits.
- *Cannellini*	- *Arugula* (25)	- *Amaranth* (100)	Mix things up for you satiation, e.g. cherry tomatoes
- *Chicken* - baked, grill/ broil, poached, sautéed, steamed	- *Asparagus* (23)	- *Angel Hair Pasta* (152)	and mozzarella, dark chocolate and nuts, celery and cheese, cottage cheese and flax seeds, sliced apple and peanut butter, strawberries and dark chocolate, etc.
	- *Berries* - blue, straw, black, red, etc.	- *Banana* (90)	
	- *Broccoli* (35)	- *Barley* (125)	
	- *Brussel Sprouts* (36)	- *Basmati Rice* (130)	
- *Cheese* (if you like a lot of cheese aim for low calorie varieties. Cottage cheese is the best as far as the ratio of protein to fat is concerned)	- *Cabbage* (23)	- *Black Beans* (132)	- *Canned Tuna*
	- *Cantalope* (34)	- *Black Eyed Peas* (116)	- *Celery*
	- *Cauliflower* (23)	- *Brown Rice* (110)	- *Cheese* (careful with fat)
	- *Celery* (18)	- *Buckwheat* (93)	- *Cherry Tomatoes*
	- *Collard* (32)	- *Bulgur* (83)	- *Chewing Gum* - sugar free
- *Egg Whites* - buy in bulk and treat them as you would an egg.	- *Cranberry* (46)	- *Butternut Squash* (40)	- *Dark Chocolate* 70-85%
	- *Cucumber* (15)	- *Carrots* (35)	cocoa
		- *Cereal* (~400)	
		- *Corn* (98)	

BEAT YOUR WEIGHT BEAT YOUR FAT

- *Fish* - baked, grilled,/ broiled, microwaved, poached, sous vide, steamed. Care with the fat, e.g. anchovy, catfish, eel, herring, mackerel, salmon, sardine, trout, whitefish.
- *Greek Yoghurt*
- *High Protein Bread-* (10g+ per slice. Fry with egg whites for even more. Works well with added fruit)
- *Lamb* - baked, braised, grilled/broiled, pan-fried, roast, steamed
- *Legumes* - care with calories.
- *Milk* (high protein and low fat , or substitute like almond, rice, etc)
- *Organ Meats* (liver, kidney, etc)
- *Pork* - braised, grill, pan-fry
- *Protein Powder* (100–150 cal/30g serving). Get creative: bars, cookies, ice-cream, milkshake, nuggets, pancakes, etc.
- *Salad* - chicken, cottage cheese, egg, tuna
- *Shellfish*
- *Soya*

- *Edamame* (120). Care with calories.
- *Eggplant* (35)
- *Fennel* (31)
- *Fruit* (any)
- *Ginger* unsweetened (80)
- *Grapefruit* (42)
- *Grapes* (70)
- *Kale* (28)
- *Leeks* (30)
- *Lettuce* (17)
- *Mango* (60)
- *Mushrooms* (28)
- *Nectarine* (45)
- *Onions* (43)
- *Orange* (50)
- *Papaya* (43)
- *Peach* (40)
- *Pear* (57)
- *Peppers* (28)
- *Pickles (care with sugar)*
- *Plum* (45)
- *Pomegranate* (83)
- *Pumpkin* (20)
- *Rabe* (22)
- *Radish* (16)
- *Salsa* (28)
- *Scallions* (32)
- *Spinach* (23)
- *Sprouts* (23)
- *Squash* (23)
- *Tangerine* (53)
- *Tomatoes* (18)

- *Couscous* (114)
- *Garlic* (150)
- *Hash-Browns* (273)
- *Jasmine Rice* (130)
- *Kidney Beans* (128)
- *Lima Beans* (115)
- *Linguine* (160)
- *Long Grain Rice* (130)
- *Millet* (120)
- *Navy Beans* (140)
- *Oats* (375)
- *Oatmeal* unsweetened (72)
- *Parsnips* (72)
- *Pasta* (157).
- *Pasta Salad*
- *Peas* (85)
- *Potatoes* (95)
- *Pretzels* (390)
- *Quinoa* (120)
- *Rice* (130)
- *Ritz Crackers* (480)
- *Rye* (250)
- *Saltines* (430)
- *Spaghetti* (150)
- *Spelt* (125)
- *Sweetcorn* (95)
- *Sweet Potato* (90)
- *Triticale* (335)

- *Edamame.* Care with calories.
- *Fruits (fresh)*
- *Fruits (frozen)* bananas (peeled) and grapes work particularly well
- *Greek Yoghurt*
- *Greek Yoghurt Ice-Cream Bars*
- *High Fibre Cereal* (Shredded wheat, All-Bran, etc)
- *Hummus* (low calorie)
- *Jerky* - Care with the sugary ones.
- *Kale*
- *Kettle Corn*
- *Milk* (high protein or substitute like almond, rice, etc)
- *Nuts* (*small* handful, and no more than once/day)
- *Olives*
- *Peanut Butter* (powdered. PB2, PBfit, etc)
- *Peppers*
- *Pickled Gherkins*
- *Pomegranate*
- *Popcorn* - self-popped or *low* calorie
- **Protein Bars, cookies, ice-cream, milkshake, nuggets, pancakes, etc -** *Must be homemade.* Bought ones are often not what they seem.

	- *Turnips* (25)	- *Whole Grain* - bagels,	- *Turkey Rolls-Ups*
	- *Vegetable Soup*	barley, bread, buckwheat,	- *Vegetable Soup*
	- *Zucchini* (15)	buns, wrap, cereal (high	- *Whole Grain Crackers*
		fibre is best for satiation),	
		crackers, flour, muffin,	
		oats, pasta, pita bread (try	
		sourdough as an alternative	
		to wholegrain), rice.	
		- *Zita* (156)	

OMEGA-3

There are 3 types of omega-3: ALA, EPA, and DHA. The body wants all of them. ALA can be converted to EPA and DHA in the body, but not efficiently, so whilst I've listed a number of items here it should be noted that only the fish has the EPA + DHA. The others are ALA. Use supplements if you don't like fish (wild and oily is best) and can afford it (take algae supplements if vegan).

- *Algal Oil*	- *Eggs*	- *Navy Beans*	- *Soybeans*
- *Anchovies*	- *Grape Leaves*	- *Oysters*	- *Spearmint*
- *Avocado*	- *Halibut*	- *Purslane*	- *Spinach*
- *Basil*	- *Herring*	- *Salmon*	- *Tofu*
- *Broccoli*	- *Kale*	- *Sardines*	- *Tuna*
- *Brussel Sprouts*	- *Kiwi*	- *Scallops*	- *Walnuts*
- *Cauliflower*	- *Leafy Greens*	- *Seaweed*	- *Winter Squash*
- *Caviar*	- *Mackerel*	- *Shrimp*	
- *Dairy*	- *Natto*	- *Snapper*	

TO BOOST HDL (GOOD CHOLESTEROL)

- *Increase mono-unsaturated fat intake.*

- *Cranberry Juice*

- *Cut out trans fats*

- *Decrease saturated fat*

- *Reduce body fat levels*

- *Increase physical activity* - 150+ minutes/week (moderate), 75+ minutes/week (vigorous). These are minimums.

OUR GUT BACTERIA AND BIOTICS

There's lots of claims here but little is entirely clear as far as any of the extreme health claims go —although veggies and fruits, as well as whole foods in general, are certainly protective (due most likely to the vitamins, minerals, and nutrient content)—but looking into gut bacteria means we bump into the *biotics* term, where there's *pro*biotics (for replenishing our bacteria), *pre*biotics (for feeding them), and then *anti*biotics (for killing them). Collectively these are known as *syn*biotics. There's also *post*biotics, which are compounds (like *short-chain fatty acids*) generated by our gut bacteria after feeding them with prebiotics.

Fibre makes it to our gut bacteria and can therefore feed them (prebiotic), and feeding our gut bacteria with food they like appears to create a craving for these types of food, and craving fibre is a particularly beneficial thing when pursuing fat loss because it's nutritional and non-fattening/calorie sparing. Feeding our good gut bacteria may also help those whose obesity has resulted in their satiety mechanism having gone somewhat awry.

Eating probiotics looks to support replenishment of our good gut bacteria and help them set up shop and protect us from other, damaging, opportunistic bacteria.[1] *Any fermented foods* are probiotic in nature (although not if pickled with vinegar), whereas *any food that reaches the gut bacteria* in the first place is a prebiotic (this mostly means fibre and resistant starch). Probiotics can also be obtained through concentrated means, such as capsules and dedicated drinks.

---

[1] In respect of bowel or digestion problems then about 4 weeks of a probiotic to see if it's helping. If not, change it to another probiotic.

There are many bacteria, and many of which whose effects on us are unknown, but the few that have been given a seal of approval, are beneficial, and that we can purposefully and directly get into our diet are *lactobacilli, bifidobacteria,* and *saccharomyces boulardii* (which is a yeast, and not a bacteria, so they're immune to antibiotics). *Akkermansia muciniphilia* is also a bacterium worthy of mention due to its association with leanness, but targeting this isn't so straight forward (although a reduction in fat and an increase in fibre would appear to promote it, particularly fibre rich in *polyphenol*—see below). *Faecalibacterium* is another, and again this isn't so straight forward to get (and dies in the air so we can't supplement for it).

Stuff like this is again additional bricks in our fat loss program to help us, not magic wands, and *your diet always comes first* (and just dropping fat and exercising also appears to shift the obese bacterial ratios into the lean ratios, which would again indicate fat loss, not gut bacteria, as the main driver of improved physical health).

Anyway, the following lists have all of the above bacteria in mind, but just because something is not in the lists doesn't mean it doesn't have benefits (e.g. natto), as it's worth repeating (and remembering) that *any fermented food* is probiotic, and *any food that reaches the gut bacteria* is prebiotic.

PROBIOTICS

- Brined Olives
- Cucumbers (fermented/pickled in salt and water)
- Dark chocolate
- Kefir
- Kimchi
- Kombucha
- Miso soup
- Gherkins
- Sauerkraut
- Soy milk
- Tempeh
- Yoghurt (particularly Greek)

FOR POLYPHENOL

- Black Beans
- Cloves
- Cocoa and Dark Chocolate
- Fruit (apples, berries, cherries, currents, grapes, plums)
- Nuts (almonds, hazelnuts, pecans, walnuts)
- Red Onions
- Red Wine
- Soy
- Spinach
- Tea (black and green)

PREBIOTICS

Prebiotics are foods eaten and liked by our good gut bacteria (and unusable by bad bacteria). Feeding our good gut bacteria results is them growing in power and gaining the upper hand in our gut. Lack of good gut bacteria is being linked to many conditions, such as diabetes, inflammation, metabolic syndrome, cardio vascular disease, depression and autoimmune diseases, to name only a few. Kinda scary. So alas, one last time for posterity, *eat more fibre.*

- Antichokes
- Apples
- Asparagus
- Bananas (the more green the better)
- Barley
- Cheese (cheddar, cottage, mozzarella. Look on the label for live and active cultures)
- Chicory Root
- Chives
- Endive leaves
- Garlic

- Leeks
- Legumes (plants in the pea family, like beans, chickpeas, kidney beans, lentils, lima beans, peanuts, peas, soybeans, etc)
- Lettuce
- Oats & Grains
- Onions
- Resistant Starch (pasta, rice, potato, etc., that's been cooked and then allowed to cool)
- Salsify
- Seaweed
- Shallots

Letter From Ian

I want to say a huge thank you for choosing to read *Beat Your Weight*, including getting all the way to the end! I very much hope it has the answer you're looking for. Even if it didn't and you don't actually see it aligning with your lifestyle, I hope it's given you some worthy insight into how to approach your dieting, fat loss and/or nutrition goals in the future.

If you did enjoy it, and especially if it has the answer you're looking for, I would be forever grateful if you'd take a minute to write a review. I'd love to hear what you think, even how it could be made even better if you think I've short-changed coverage of a particular topic in your view.

Reviews greatly help indie authors such as myself, as well as helping other readers discover work for the first time. Amazon reviews are particularly helpful. You could even recommend or lend it to a friend or family member who you think this may be what they're looking for themselves.

Whatever you do, all the best.

Ian

References

AUTHOR NOTE

"Extra Calories Cause Weight Gain—But How Much?" doi.org/10.1001/jama.2009.1912

INTRODUCTION

"Body-mass index and all-cause mortality: individual-participant-data meta-analysis of 239 prospective studies in four continents" doi.org/10.1016/S0140-6736(16)30175-1

"The Obesity Paradox: Fact or Fiction?" doi.org/10.1016/j.amjcard.2006.04.039

"The Obese Without Cardiometabolic Risk Factor Clustering and the Normal Weight With Cardiometabolic Risk Factor Clustering" doi.org/10.1001/archinte.168.15.1617

"The long-term prognosis of cardiovascular disease and all-cause mortality for metabolically healthy obesity: a systematic review and meta-analysis" doi.org/10.1136/jech-2015-206948

"Metabolically healthy obesity and risk of cardiovascular disease, cancer, and all-cause and cause-specific mortality: a protocol for a systematic review and meta-analysis of prospective studies" dx.doi.org/10.1136%2Fbmjopen-2019-032742/

"Metabolically Healthy Obesity" doi.org/10.1210/endrev/bnaa004

"Obesity Paradox and Cardiorespiratory Fitness in 12,417 Male Veterans Aged 40 to 70 Years" doi.org/10.4065/mcp.2009.0562

"*How Fat Works*" - Harvard University Press (2009). Philip A. Wood

"The Medical Risks of Obesity" ncbi.nlm.nih.gov/pmc/articles/PMC2879283/

"New genetic loci link adipose and insulin biology to body fat distribution" ncbi.nlm.nih.gov/pmc/articles/PMC4338562/

"Differential effect of subcutaneous abdominal and visceral adipose tissue on cardiometabolic risk" doi.org/10.1515/hmb-ci-2018-0014

"Endometrial Cancer, Obesity, and Body Fat Distribution" cancerres.aacrjournals.org/content/canres/51/2/568.full.pdf

"Transplantation of non-visceral fat to the visceral cavity improves glucose tolerance in mice: investigation of hepatic lipids and insulin sensitivity" dx.doi.org/10.1007%2Fs00125-011-2259-5/

"Cellular mechanism of insulin resistance in nonalcoholic fatty liver disease" doi.org/10.1073/pnas.1113359108

"About Diabetes" tinyurl.com/y2j4cjmq

"Adipose tissue inflammation in obesity and metabolic syndrome" tinyurl.com/y4eqb5by

"Adipose tissue inflammation in obesity: a metabolic or immune response?" pubmed.ncbi.nlm.nih.gov/28843953/

"Obesity-induced inflammatory changes in adipose tissue" doi.org/10.1172/JCI20514

"Contribution of adipose tissue inflammation to the development of type 2 diabetes mellitus" ncbi.nlm.nih.gov/pmc/articles/PMC6557583/

"Adipose cell size: importance in health and disease" doi.org/10.1152/ajpregu.00257.2017

"Adipose tissue expandability and the metabolic syndrome" ncbi.nlm.nih.gov/pmc/articles/PMC2474894/

"Impaired Adipose Tissue Expandability and Lipogenic Capacities as Ones of the Main Causes of Metabolic Disorders" dx.doi.org/10.1155%2F2015%2F970375

"Guideline for the Management of Overweight and Obesity in Adults" doi.org/10.1161/01.cir.0000437739.71477.ee

"Energy balance and obesity: what are the main drivers?" dx.doi.org/10.1007%2Fs10552-017-0869-z

"OECD Health Statistics 2020" stats.oecd.org/Index.aspx?ThemeTreeId=9

"Adult Obesity Facts" tinyurl.com/yxqox6e2

"Prevalence of Obesity and Severe Obesity Among Adults: United States, 2017–2018" tinyurl.com/qudcl8x

"What share of adults are obese/overweight?" www.ourworldindata.org/obesity#what-share-of-adults-are-overweight

"The Role of Adipose Tissue and Adipokines in Obesity-Related Inflammatory Diseases" doi.org/10.1155/2010/802078

"Obesity and Its Metabolic Complications: The Role of Adipokines and the Relationship between Obesity, Inflammation, Insulin Resistance, Dyslipidemia and Nonalcoholic Fatty Liver Disease" ncbi.nlm.nih.gov/pmc/articles/PMC4013623/

THE PROBLEMS

I would like to thank Dr Layne Norton who brought liraglutide to my attention. This made me take a deep dive into sugar and insulin resulting in an extensive overhaul to my original theory of it. Layne Norton's website is www.biolayne.com

"A map of human genome variation from population-scale sequencing" dx.doi.org/10.1038%2Fnature09534

"A global reference for human genetic variation" dx.doi.org/10.1038%2Fnature15393

"Energy balance and obesity: what are the main drivers?" dx.doi.org/10.1007%2Fs10552-017-0869-z

GETTING FUEL

"Biochemical, Physiological, and Molecular Aspects of Human Nutrition, 3rd Edition" - Saunders (2012). Martha Stipanuk, Marie Caudill.

"How Fat Works" - Harvard University Press (2009). Philip A. Wood

A PROPOSED PROBLEM

"How Fat Works" - Harvard University Press (2009). Philip A. Wood

"The Carbohydrate-Insulin Model of Obesity: Beyond 'Calories In, Calories Out'" doi.org/10.1001/jamainternmed.2018.2933

"Regulation of Triglyceride Metabolism. IV. Hormonal regulation of lipolysis in adipose tissue" doi.org/10.1152/ajpgi.00554.2006

"Mechanisms of nutritional and hormonal regulation of lipogenesis" doi.org/10.1093/embo-reports/kve071

An insulin index of foods: the insulin demand generated by 1000-kJ portions of common foods" doi.org/10.1093/ajcn/66.5.1264

"Insulinotropic Effects of Whey: Mechanisms of Action, Recent Clinical Trials, and Clinical Applications" doi.org/10.1159/000448665

"Liraglutide for weight management: a critical review of the evidence" onlinelibrary.wiley.com/doi/full/10.1002/osp4.84

"Liraglutide With Insulin Improves Glycemic Control in Type 1 Diabetes, Without More Hypoglycemia" tinyurl.com/y5l3unvn

"Liraglutide as an Additional Treatment to Insulin in Patients with Type 1 Diabetes Mellitus—A 52-Week Randomized Double-Blinded Placebo-Controlled Clinical Trial" doi.org/10.2337/db18-3-LB

"A Randomized, Controlled Trial of 3.0 mg of Liraglutide in Weight Management" doi.org/10.1056/nejmoa1411892

"Circulating FGF21 in humans is potently induced by short term overfeeding of carbohydrates" ncbi.nlm.nih.gov/pmc/articles/PMC5220397/

"Fibroblast Growth Factor 21: A Versatile Regulator of Metabolic Homeostasis" ncbi.nlm.nih.gov/pmc/articles/PMC6964258/

"Going Back to the Biology of FGF21: New Insights" doi.org/10.1016/j.tem.2019.05.007

ENERGY BALANCE

"Biochemical, Physiological, and Molecular Aspects of Human Nutrition, 3rd Edition" - Saunders (2012). Martha Stipanuk, Marie Caudill

"Dietary modifications for weight loss and weight loss maintenance" doi.org/10.1016/j.metabol.2019.01.001

"The Carbohydrate-Insulin Model of Obesity: Beyond 'Calories In, Calories Out'" doi.org/10.1001/jamainternmed.2018.2933

"Pancreatic signals controlling food intake; insulin, glucagon and amylin" doi.org/10.1098/rstb.2006.1858

"Relationship between body fat mass and free fatty acid kinetics in men and women" doi.org/10.1038/oby.2009.224

SUGAR

"The Case Against Sugar" - Portobello Books (2017). Gary Taubes

REFERENCES

"Reward, dopamine and the control of food intake: implications for obesity" ncbi.nlm.nih.gov/pmc/articles/PMC3124340/

"Excessive Consumption of Sugar: an Insatiable Drive for Reward" doi.org/10.1007/s13668-019-0270-5

"Frontostriatal and behavioral adaptations to daily sugar-sweetened beverage intake: a randomized controlled trial" doi.org/10.3945/ajcn.116.140145

"The Carbohydrate-Insulin Model of Obesity: Beyond 'Calories In, Calories Out'" doi.org/10.1001/jamainternmed.2018.2933

"Long-term Effects of a Very Low-Carbohydrate Diet and a Low-Fat Diet on Mood and Cognitive Function" doi.org/10.1001/archinternmed.2009.329

"Modification of immune responses to exercise by carbohydrate, glutamine and anti-oxidant supplements" doi.org/10.1111/j.1440-1711.2000.t01-6-.x

"Diet-hormone interactions: protein/carbohydrate ratio alters reciprocally the plasma levels of testosterone and cortisol and their respective binding globulins in man" pubmed.ncbi.nlm.nih.gov/3573976/

"Influence of dietary carbohydrate intake on the free testosterone: cortisol ratio responses to short-term intensive exercise training" link.springer.com/article/10.1007/s00421-009-1220-5

"Dietary-induced alterations in thyroid hormone metabolism during overnutrition" doi.org/10.1172/JCI109590

"Isocaloric carbohydrate deprivation induces protein catabolism despite a low T3-syndrome in healthy men" doi.org/10.1046/j.1365-2265.2001.01158.x

THE REAL PROBLEM

"Carbohydrate bioavailability" doi.org/10.1079/BJN20051457

"Postprandial energy expenditure in whole-food and processed-food meals: implications for daily energy expenditure" doi.org/10.3402/fnr.v54i0.5144

"Substituting whole grains for refined grains in a 6-wk randomized trial favorably affects energy-balance metrics in healthy men and postmenopausal women" doi.org/10.3945/ajcn.116.139683

"Oatmeal particle size alters glycemic index but not as a function of gastric emptying rate" doi.org/10.1152/ajpgi.00005.2017

"Particle size, satiety and the glycaemic response" pubmed.ncbi.nlm.nih.gov/7956991/

"The Thermic Effect of Food: A Review" doi.org/10.1080/07315724.2018.1552544

"Greater Whole-Grain Intake Is Associated with Lower Risk of Type 2 Diabetes, Cardiovascular Disease, and Weight Gain" doi.org/10.3945/jn.111.155325

"Substituting whole grain for refined grain: what is needed to strengthen the scientific evidence for health outcomes?" doi.org/10.3945/ajcn.117.152496

"Metabolic effects of dietary fiber consumption and prevention of diabetes" doi.org/10.1093/jn/138.3.439

"Dietary fiber and body weight" doi.org/10.1016/j.nut.2004.08.018

"Dietary Fiber and Metabolic Syndrome: A Meta-Analysis and Review of Related Mechanisms" doi.org/10.3390/nu10010024

"Impact of dietary fiber intake on glycemic control, cardiovascular risk factors and chronic kidney disease in Japanese patients with type 2 diabetes mellitus: the Fukuoka Diabetes Registry" dx.doi.org/10.1186%2F1475-2891-12-159

"Dietary fibre and whole grains in diabetes management: Systematic review and meta-analyses" doi.org/10.1371/journal.pmed.1003053

"Dietary fibre and incidence of type 2 diabetes in eight European countries" dx.doi.org/10.1007%2Fs00125-015-3585-9

"Fuel not fun: reinterpreting attenuated brain responses to reward in obesity" ncbi.nlm.nih.gov/pmc/articles/PMC4971522/

"Reward, dopamine and the control of food intake: implications for obesity" ncbi.nlm.nih.gov/pmc/articles/PMC3124340/

"Excessive Consumption of Sugar: an Insatiable Drive for Reward" doi.org/10.1007/s13668-019-0270-5

THE 4-STEP PROCESS OF OBESITY

"Reward, dopamine and the control of food intake: implications for obesity" ncbi.nlm.nih.gov/pmc/articles/PMC3124340/

"Excessive Consumption of Sugar: an Insatiable Drive for Reward" doi.org/10.1007/s13668-019-0270-5

"Frontostriatal and behavioral adaptations to daily sugar-sweetened beverage intake: a randomized controlled trial" doi.org/10.3945/ajcn.116.140145

"Variety and hyperpalatability: are they promoting addictive overeating?" doi.org/10.3945/ajcn.111.020164

THE FIX

"Diet in Early Homo: A Review of the Evidence and a New Model of Adaptive Versatility" tinyurl.com/y4w5v9xn

"Paleofantasy: What Evolution Really Tells Us about Sex, Diet, and How We Live" - W. W. Norton & Company (2013). Marlene Zuk

"What is the Mechanism Behind Weight Loss Maintenance with Gastric Bypass?" doi.org/10.1007/s13679-015-0158-7

"Long term gluten consumption in adults without celiac disease and risk of coronary heart disease: prospective cohort study" dx.doi.org/10.1136/bmj.j1892

"Impact of diet on breast cancer risk" doi.org/10.1097/GCO.0b013e32831d7f22

"Diet and breast cancer" doi.org/10.1002/cncr.22654

"Independent Introduction of Two Lactase-Persistence Alleles into Human Populations Reflects Different History of Adaptation to Milk Culture" doi.org/10.1016/j.ajhg.2007.09.012

"Evolution of lactase persistence: an example of human niche construction" doi.org/10.1098/rstb.2010.0268

"Convergent adaptation of human lactase persistence in Africa and Europe" ncbi.nlm.nih.gov/pmc/articles/PMC2672153/

WHAT DIETS DO RIGHT

"How Fat Works" - Harvard University Press (2009). Philip A. Wood

THE FIX

"Effect of Low-Fat vs Low-Carbohydrate Diet on 12-Month Weight Loss in Overweight Adults and the Association With Genotype Pattern or Insulin Secretion" doi.org/10.1001/jama.2018.0245

"Association of Low-Carbohydrate and Low-Fat Diets With Mortality Among US Adults" doi.org/10.1001/jamainternmed.2019.6980

"Effects Of Dietary Protein On The Composition Of Weight Loss In Post-Menopausal Women" ncbi.nlm.nih.gov/pmc/articles/PMC3629809/

"Effect of an isocaloric diet containing fiber-enriched flour on anthropometric and biochemical parameters in healthy non-obese non-diabetic subjects" doi.org/10.3164/jcbn.14-133

"An Overview of the Effects of Dietary Fiber on Gastrointestinal Transit" pediatrics.aappublications.org/content/96/5/997

"Ratios of soluble and insoluble dietary fibers on satiety and energy intake in overweight pre- and postmenopausal women" dx.doi.org/10.3233%2FNHA-160018

"Gut microbiota fermentation of prebiotics increases satietogenic and incretin gut peptide production with consequences for appetite sensation and glucose response after a meal" doi.org/10.3945/ajcn.2009.28095

"Maintenance of energy expenditure on high-protein vs. high-carbohydrate diets at a constant body weight may prevent a positive energy balance" doi.org/10.1016/j.clnu.2014.10.007

"The Energy Costs of Protein Metabolism" ncbi.nlm.nih.gov/books/NBK224633/

"Protein quantity and quality at levels above the RDA improves adult weight loss" doi.org/10.1080/07315724.2004.10719435

"A Moderate-Protein Diet Produces Sustained Weight Loss and Long-Term Changes in Body Composition and Blood Lipids in Obese Adults" doi.org/10.3945/jn.108.099440

"A high-protein diet induces sustained reductions in appetite, ad libitum caloric intake, and body weight despite compensatory changes in diurnal plasma leptin and ghrelin concentrations" doi.org/10.1093/ajcn/82.1.41

"Lean Mass Loss Is Associated with Low Protein Intake during Dietary-Induced Weight Loss in Postmenopausal Women" ncbi.nlm.nih.gov/pmc/articles/PMC3665330/

"Calorie restriction accelerates the catabolism of lean body mass during 2 wk of bed rest" doi.org/10.1093/ajcn/86.2.366

"Dietary Protein and Exercise Have Additive Effects on Body Composition during Weight Loss in Adult Women" doi.org/10.1093/jn/135.8.1903

"Diet induced thermogenesis" hdx.doi.org/10.1186%2F1743-7075-1-5

"Thermic effect of food, exercise, and total energy expenditure in active females" tinyurl.com/yygswahx

"The Effect of Dietary Protein on Weight Loss, Satiety, and Appetite Hormone" www.actascientific.com/ASNH/pdf/ASNH-03-0207.pdf

"Effect of high-protein breakfast meal on within-day appetite hormones: Peptide YY, glucagon like peptide-1 in adults" doi.org/10.1016/j.yclnex.2019.09.002

"Increased Protein Intake Reduces Lean Body Mass Loss during Weight Loss in Athletes" doi.org/10.1249/MSS.0b013e3181b2ef8e

"A systematic review of dietary protein during caloric restriction in resistance trained lean athletes: a case for higher intakes" tinyurl.com/yauek6lz

"A high proportion of leucine is required for optimal stimulation of the rate of muscle protein synthesis by essential amino acids in the elderly" doi.org/10.1152/ajpendo.00488.2005

SATIATION

"Putting the Balance Back in Diet" doi.org/10.1016/j.cell.2015.02.033

"Protein, weight management, and satiety" doi.org/10.1093/ajcn/87.5.1558S

"Divergent effects of central melanocortin signalling on fat and sucrose preference in humans" dx.doi.org/10.1038%2Fncomms13055

REFERENCES

"The Effect of Dietary Protein on Weight Loss, Satiety, and Appetite Hormone" www.actascientific.com/ASNH/pdf/ASNH-03-0207.pdf

"Effect of high-protein breakfast meal on within-day appetite hormones: Peptide YY, glucagon like peptide-1 in adults" doi.org/10.1016/j.yclnex.2019.09.002

STARCH & FAT

"*How Fat Works*" - Harvard University Press (2009). Philip A. Wood

"Calorie for calorie, dietary fat restriction results in more body fat loss than carbohydrate restriction in people with obesity" doi.org/10.1016/j.cmet.2015.07.021

"A systematic review of the effect of dietary saturated and polyunsaturated fat on heart disease" doi.org/10.1016/j.numecd.2017.10.010

"Three Weeks on a High-Fat Diet Increases Intrahepatic Lipid Accumulation and Decreases Metabolic Flexibility in Healthy Overweight Men" doi.org/10.1210/jc.2010-2243

"Influence of dietary macronutrients on liver fat accumulation and metabolism" tinyurl.com/y3r6cyl2

"Poly is more Effective than Mono - Unsaturated Fat For dietary management IN the Metabolic Syndrome" ncbi.nlm.nih.gov/pmc/articles/PMC5010036/

"No need to avoid healthy omega-6 fats" tinyurl.com/yxv9lmwl

"The Omega-6:Omega-3 ratio: A critical appraisal and possible successor" tinyurl.com/y6ss3t82

"Omega-6 fatty acids and inflammation" tinyurl.com/yypaxv32

"An Increase in the Omega-6/Omega-3 Fatty Acid Ratio Increases the Risk for Obesity" dx.doi.org/10.3390%2Fnu8030128

"Omega-6 fats for the primary and secondary prevention of cardiovascular disease" doi.org/10.1002/14651858.CD011094.pub3

"Factors influencing variation in basal metabolic rate include fat-free mass, fat mass, age, and circulating thyroxine but not sex, circulating leptin, or triiodothyronine" doi.org/10.1093/ajcn/82.5.941

THE METHOD

It's been queried that the method proposed is an adaption to MyPlate (www.choosemyplate.gov/resources/myplate-graphic-resources), but really the method proposed is reasoned from the benefits of protein and fibre as elucidated on in the preceding chapters.

HOW TO NOT FAIL

"Long-term weight loss maintenance in the United States" dx.doi.org/10.1038%2Fijo.2010.94

"Does dieting make you fat? A twin study" doi.org/10.1038/ijo.2011.160

"How dieting makes some fatter: from a perspective of human body composition autoregulation" doi.org/10.1017/S0029665112000225

"Persistent metabolic adaptation 6 years after The Biggest Loser competition" ncbi.nlm.nih.gov/pmc/articles/PMC4989512/

"Physiological adaptations to weight loss and factors favouring weight regain" doi.org/10.1038/ijo.2015.59

"Consequences of Weight Cycling: An Increase in Disease Risk?" ncbi.nlm.nih.gov/pmc/articles/PMC4241770/

"Biology's response to dieting: the impetus for weight regain" doi.org/10.1152/ajpregu.00755.2010

"Effect of caloric restriction and dietary composition on serum T3 and Reverse T3 in man" doi.org/10.1210/jcem-42-1-197

"Metabolic adaptations to weight loss" ncbi.nlm.nih.gov/pmc/articles/PMC6086582/

"Weight-loss attempts and risk of major weight gain: a prospective study in Finnish adults" doi.org/10.1093/ajcn/70.6.965

"Metabolic Slowing with Massive Weight Loss despite Preservation of Fat-Free Mass" doi.org/10.1210/jc.2012-1444

"Moderate Weight Loss Is Sufficient to Affect Thyroid Hormone Homeostasis and Inhibit Its Peripheral Conversion" ncbi.nlm.nih.gov/pmc/articles/PMC3887425/

"The role for adipose tissue in weight regain after weight loss" doi.org/10.1111/obr.12255

"Metabolic adaptation following massive weight loss is related to the degree of energy imbalance and changes in circulating leptin" doi.org/10.1002/oby.20900

"Changes in Energy Expenditure Resulting from Altered Body Weight" doi.org/10.1056/NEJM199503093321001

"Greater than predicted decrease in energy expenditure during exercise after body weight loss in obese men" doi.org/10.1042/CS20020252

"Peptide YY levels are decreased by fasting and elevated following caloric intake but are not regulated by leptin" doi.org/10.1007/s00125-005-0041-2

"Twenty-four-hour Ghrelin Is Elevated after Calorie Restriction and Exercise Training in Non-obese Women" doi.org/10.1038/oby.2007.542

"Weight loss increases circulating levels of ghrelin in human obesity" doi.org/10.1046/j.0300-0664.2001.01456.x

"Hypothalamic Sites of Leptin Action Linking Metabolism and Reproduction" doi.org/10.1159/000322472

"Long-term persistence of adaptive thermogenesis in subjects who have maintained a reduced body weight" doi.org/10.1093/ajcn/88.4.906

"Adaptive changes in energy expenditure during refeeding following low-calorie intake: evidence for a specific metabolic component favoring fat storage" doi.org/10.1093/ajcn/52.3.415

"Effect of weight reduction on resting energy expenditure, substrate utilization, and the thermic effect of food in moderately obese women" tinyurl.com/y3b3effb

"Exposure to endocrine-disrupting chemicals and anthropometric measures of obesity: a systematic review and meta-analysis" dx.doi.org/10.1136%2Fbmjopen-2019-033509

"Adverse effects of weight loss: Are persistent organic pollutants a potential culprit?" doi.org/10.1016/j.diabet.2016.05.009

"Persistent organic pollutants & obesity: potential mechanisms for breast cancer promotion?" doi.org/10.1530/ERC-14-0411

"Persistent organic pollutants in adipose tissue should be considered in obesity research" doi.org/10.1111/obr.12481

*A potential saving grace: "*No consistent evidence of a disproportionately low resting energy expenditure in long-term successful weight-loss maintainers" doi.org/10.1093/ajcn/nqy179

HOW TO GO SLOW

"Metabolic adaptation following massive weight loss is related to the degree of energy imbalance and changes in circulating leptin" doi.org/10.1002/oby.20900

"Long-term efficacy of dietary treatment of obesity: a systematic review of studies published between 1931 and 1999" doi.org/10.1046/j.1467-789x.2000.00019.x

THE TWO-TYPES

On Categories: This is just my personal observation. It could also be appropriate to include more categories for eating disorders, but eating disorders should be addressed with professional guidance and it's probably not the time to diet any way if you suffer from one of these. The Five Steps For Success as well as point 6 of "what to do about hunger?" may be of assistance. For binge eating in particular, commit yourself to three things: 1) eating slowly, 2) regular intervals of eating (such as 3 meals and 2 snacks a day—don't intermittent fast or restrict yourself into an inevitable binge), and 3) if you do binge, then binge on fibre and lean protein, i.e. low calorie dense food, before you binge on the other stuff. That way you'll have filled yourself up some before you start on the high calorie stuff. Binge eating is still an eating disorder mind, so seeking professional help is still the best idea if you can't stop on your own.

"Nudge: Improving Decisions About Health, Wealth, and Happiness" - Penguin Books (2008) Richard H. Thaler, Cass R. Sunstein

"Portion, package or tableware size for changing selection and consumption of food, alcohol and tobacco" doi.org/10.1002/14651858.CD011045

"Automatic and Controlled Processing: Implications for Eating Behavior" doi.org/10.3390/nu12041097

STAGNATION

"Metabolic adaptation is not a major barrier to weight-loss maintenance" doi.org/10.1093/ajcn/nqaa086

FIVE STEPS FOR SUCCESS

"Long-term weight loss maintenance for obesity: a multidisciplinary approach" doi.org/10.2147/DMSO.S89836

"Attenuating the Biologic Drive for Weight Regain Following Weight Loss: Must What Goes Down Always Go Back Up?" doi.org/10.3390/nu9050468

EXERCISING CONTROL & THE POWER OF WILL

"The Hormonal Control of Food Intake" doi.org/10.1016/j.cell.2007.04.001

"Food craving in daily life: comparison of overweight and normal-weight participants with ecological momentary assessment" doi.org/10.1111/jhn.12693

"Genetic studies of body mass index yield new insights for obesity biology" ncbi.nlm.nih.gov/pmc/articles/PMC4382211/pdf/nihms-668049.pdf

"Clinical Spectrum of Obesity and Mutations in the Melanocortin 4 Receptor Gene" doi.org/10.1056/NEJMoa022050

"A Deletion in the Canine POMC Gene Is Associated with Weight and Appetite in Obesity-Prone Labrador Retriever Dogs" doi.org/10.1016/j.cmet.2016.04.012

"Successful Weight Loss Among Obese U.S. Adults" ncbi.nlm.nih.gov/pmc/articles/PMC3339766/

"Portion, package or tableware size for changing selection and consumption of food, alcohol and tobacco" doi.org/10.1002/14651858.CD011045

"The color red reduces snack food and soft drink intake" https://doi.org/10.1016/j.appet.2011.12.023

"Weight Loss and the Prevention of Weight Regain: Evaluation of a Treatment Model of Exercise Self-Regulation Generalizing to Controlled Eating" doi.org/10.7812/TPP/15-146

REFERENCES

"Dietary and physical activity behaviors among adults successful at weight loss maintenance" doi.org/10.1186/1479-5868-3-17

"Energy Intake and Exercise as Determinants of Brain Health and Vulnerability to Injury and Disease" doi.org/10.1016/j.cmet.2012.08.012

"*Skeletal Tissue Mechanics*" - Springer (2015). Martin, R.B., Burr, D.B., Sharkey, N.A., Fyhrie, D.P.

"Skeletal Muscle Hypertrophy Following Resistance Training Is Accompanied by a Fiber Type–Specific Increase in Satellite Cell Content in Elderly Men" doi.org/10.1093/gerona/gln050

"Skeletal Function and Form: Mechanobiology of Skeletal Development, Aging, and Regeneration" tinyurl.com/y6cd2fk4

BE MINDFUL

"What Matters in Weight Loss? An In-Depth Analysis of Self-Monitoring" doi.org/10.2196/jmir.7457

EYES ON THE PRIZE

"Eyes on the prize: The longitudinal benefits of goal focus on progress toward a weight loss goal" ncbi.nlm.nih.gov/pmc/articles/PMC3104274/

"The Biggest Loser Thinks Long-Term: Recency as a Predictor of Success in Weight Management" ncbi.nlm.nih.gov/pmc/articles/PMC4672063/

"Dieting and the self-control of eating in everyday environments: An experience sampling study" ncbi.nlm.nih.gov/pmc/articles/PMC3784634/

EXERCISE

"Exercise in weight management of obesity" pubmed.ncbi.nlm.nih.gov/11570117

"Is regular exercise an effective strategy for weight loss maintenance?" ncbi.nlm.nih.gov/pmc/articles/PMC5929468/

"A decrease in physical activity affects appetite, energy, and nutrient balance in lean men feeding ad libitum" doi.org/10.1093/ajcn/79.1.62

"Increasing energy flux to decrease the biological drive toward weight regain after weight loss – A proof-of-concept pilot study" pubmed.ncbi.nlm.nih.gov/28531421/

Recent advances in understanding resistance exercise training-induced skeletal muscle hypertrophy in humans" dx.doi.org/10.12688%2Ff1000research.21588.1

"Preserving Healthy Muscle during Weight Loss" doi.org/10.3945/an.116.014506

"Reversal of type 2 diabetes: normalisation of beta cell function in association with decreased pancreas and liver triacylglycerol" doi.org/10.1007/s00125-011-2204-7

"Aerobic Exercise Increases Peripheral and Hepatic Insulin Sensitivity in Sedentary Adolescents" doi.org/10.1210/jc.2009-1379

"Metabolic adaptation to weight loss: implications for the athlete" doi.org/10.1186/1550-2783-11-7

"Association between muscular strength and mortality in men: prospective cohort study" doi.org/10.1136/bmj.a439

"The Effects of Exercise on Food Intake and Hunger: Relationship with Acylated Ghrelin and Leptin" ncbi.nlm.nih.gov/pmc/articles/PMC3761859/

"Exercise reduces appetite and traffics excess nutrients away from energetically efficient pathways of lipid deposition during the early stages of weight regain" doi.org/10.1152/ajpregu.00212.2011

"Effects of Exercise Modality on Insulin Resistance and Ectopic Fat in Adolescents with Overweight and Obesity: A Randomized Clinical Trial" doi.org/10.1016/j.jpeds.2018.10.059

"Effect of exercise intensity and volume on persistence of insulin sensitivity during training cessation" doi.org/10.1152/japplphysiol.91262.2008

"Skeletal muscle and beyond: the role of exercise as a mediator of systemic mitochondrial biogenesis" doi.org/10.1139/h11-076

"Skeletal muscle mitochondrial remodeling in exercise and diseases" doi.org/10.1038/s41422-018-0078-7

"The effect of high-intensity training on mitochondrial fat oxidation in skeletal muscle and subcutaneous adipose tissue" doi.org/10.1111/sms.12252

"Skeletal Muscle Hypertrophy Following Resistance Training Is Accompanied by a Fiber Type–Specific Increase in Satellite Cell Content in Elderly Men" doi.org/10.1093/gerona/gln050

"The Relative Benefits of Endurance and Strength Training on the Metabolic Factors and Muscle Function of People With Type 2 Diabetes Mellitus" doi.org/10.1016/j.apmr.2005.01.007

"A systematic review of dietary protein during caloric restriction in resistance trained lean athletes: a case for higher intakes" tinyurl.com/yauek6lz

"Calorie restriction accelerates the catabolism of lean body mass during 2 wk of bed rest" doi.org/10.1093/ajcn/86.2.366

"Marked Improvement in Carbohydrate and Lipid Metabolism in Diabetic Australian Aborigines After Temporary Reversion to Traditional Lifestyle" doi.org/10.2337/diab.33.6.596

"A High-Protein Diet With Resistance Exercise Training Improves Weight Loss and Body Composition in Overweight and Obese Patients With Type 2 Diabetes" doi.org/10.2337/dc09-1974

"Reduction in the Incidence of Type 2 Diabetes with Lifestyle Intervention or Metformin" doi.org/10.1056/NEJMoa012512

"The Physiology of Optimizing Health with a Focus on Exercise as Medicine" doi.org/10.1146/annurev-physiol-020518-114339

"The effect of physical activity on mortality and cardiovascular disease in 130 000 people from 17 high-income, middle-income, and low-income countries: the PURE study" doi.org/10.1016/S0140-6736(17)31634-3

"Physical Exercise Inhibits Inflammation and Microglial Activation" doi.org/10.3390/cells8070691

"Exercise Intervention Associated with Cognitive Improvement in Alzheimer's Disease" doi.org/10.1155/2018/9234105

"Physical exercise and cognitive performance in the elderly: current perspectives" ncbi.nlm.nih.gov/pmc/articles/PMC3872007/

"Exercise Prescriptions in Older Adults" aafp.org/afp/2017/0401/p425.html

"Exercise Prevents Diet-Induced Cellular Senescence in Adipose Tissue" doi.org/10.2337/db15-0291

"Physical Exercise Prevents Cellular Senescence in Circulating Leukocytes and in the Vessel Wall" doi.org/10.1161/CIRCULA-TIONAHA.109.861005

"Benefits of Exercise in the Older Population" doi.org/10.1016/j.pmr.2017.06.001

"Physical Exercise as Therapy for Frailty" ncbi.nlm.nih.gov/pmc/articles/PMC4712448/

"Exercise-Induced Neuroplasticity: A Mechanistic Model and Prospects for Promoting Plasticity" doi.org/10.1177%2F1073858418771538

"Regular exercise attenuates the metabolic drive to regain weight after long-term weight loss" doi.org/10.1152/ajpregu.00192.2009

"Chronic exercise lowers the defended body weight gain and adiposity in diet-induced obese rats" doi.org/10.1152/ajpregu.00650.2003

"Energy cost of isolated resistance exercises across low-to high-intensities" doi.org/10.1371/journal.pone.0181311

"Too much sitting – A health hazard" doi.org/10.1016/j.diabres.2012.05.020

"Sedentary behavior and health outcomes among older adults: a systematic review" doi.org/10.1186/1471-2458-14-333

COMMITTED TO CONSISTENCY

"Influence: Science and Practice" - Pearson (2008). Robert B. Cialdini

"Who's Pulling Your Strings" - McGraw-Hill (2003). Harriet B. Braiker

ENVIRONMENTAL STRESSES

"Sleep and obesity" doi.org/10.1097/MCO.0b013e3283479109

"Acute Sleep Deprivation Enhances the Brain's Response to Hedonic Food Stimuli: An fMRI Study" doi.org/10.1210/jc.2011-2759

"Sleep Restriction Enhances the Daily Rhythm of Circulating Levels of Endocannabinoid 2-Arachidonoylglycerol" doi.org/10.5665/sleep.5546

"A single night of sleep deprivation increases ghrelin levels and feelings of hunger in normal-weight healthy men" doi.org/10.1111/j.1365-2869.2008.00662.x

"Chronic stress and comfort foods: self-medication and abdominal obesity" doi.org/10.1016/j.bbi.2004.11.004

"Stress, eating and the reward system" doi.org/10.1016/j.physbeh.2007.04.011

"SnapShot: Stress and Disease" dx.doi.org/10.1016/j.cmet.2016.01.015

"The Pathogenetic Role of Cortisol in the Metabolic Syndrome: A Hypothesis" doi.org/10.1210/jc.2009-0370

"Relation between resting amygdalar activity and cardiovascular events: a longitudinal and cohort study" doi.org/10.1016/S0140-6736(16)31714-7

See here for some negative remarks on meditation: tinyurl.com/yy2l9hka

"Humor" doi.org/10.1016/j.psc.2014.08.006

"Virtuous laughter: we should teach medical learners the art of humor" doi.org/10.1186/s13054-015-0927-4

"Humor Theories and the Physiological Benefits of Laughter" tinyurl.com/yx9af5wy

"Comfort food is comforting to those most stressed: Evidence of the chronic stress response network in high stress women" ncbi.nlm.nih.gov/pmc/articles/PMC3425607/

"Childhood Obesity: Adrift in the "Limbic Triangle"" doi.org/10.1146/annurev.med.59.103106.105628

EPILOGUE

THE ONLY DIET PLAN WORTH CONSIDERING

"Changing the Energy Density of the Diet as a Strategy for Weight Management" doi.org/10.1016/j.jada.2005.02.033

"Effects of Dietary Composition During Weight Loss Maintenance: A Controlled Feeding Study" doi.org/10.1001/jama.2012.6607

REFERENCES

"Dietary adherence and weight loss success among overweight women: results from the A TO Z weight loss study" doi.org/10.1038/ijo.2008.8

"Lifestyle and cardiovascular disease in middle-aged British men: the effect of adjusting for within-person variation" doi.org/10.1093/eurheartj/ehi224

PAYING THE PRICE

"Delayed gratification in New Caledonian crows and young children: influence of reward type and visibility" doi.org/10.1007/s10071-019-01317-7

"Childhood Obesity and Delayed Gratification Behavior: A Systematic Review of Experimental Studies" doi.org/10.1016/j.jpeds.2015.10.008

"Functional and structural neuroimaging studies of delayed reward discounting in addiction: A systematic review" pubmed.ncbi.nlm.nih.gov/30652907/

TAKE ACTION

On healthy human heart beats: Calculated at 60 beats a minute for 80 years (~2.5 billion) but rounded down to make the sentence read better.

"Causes of death by category" ourworldindata.org/causes-of-death#causes-of-death-by-category

"The prevalence, metabolic risk and effects of lifestyle intervention for metabolically healthy obesity: a systematic review and meta-analysis" hdoi.org/10.1097/MD.0000000000008838

"Weight Gain as a Risk Factor for Clinical Diabetes Mellitus in Women" tinyurl.com/y2pv8uhn

"The importance of weight management in type 2 diabetes mellitus" doi.org/10.1111/ijcp.12384

"Effects on cardiovascular risk factors of weight losses limited to 5–10 %" ncbi.nlm.nih.gov/pmc/articles/PMC4987606/

"Effects of weight loss interventions for adults who are obese on mortality, cardiovascular disease, and cancer: systematic review and meta-analysis" doi.org/10.1136/bmj.j4849

"Intentional weight loss and cancer risk" dx.doi.org/10.18632%2Foncotarget.20671

"The Relationship between Metabolically Healthy Obesity and the Risk of Cardiovascular Disease: A Systematic Review and Meta-Analysis" doi.org/10.3390/jcm8081228

APPENDIX 1 - Q&A

ARE YOU SURE THIS ISN'T A DIET?

On the etymology of diet: www.etymonline.com/word/diet

YOU'RE TELLING ME TO EAT A LOT OF MEAT

"Reduction of Red and Processed Meat Intake and Cancer Mortality and Incidence" doi.org/10.7326/M19-0699

"Red Meat and Colorectal Cancer: A Quantitative Update on the State of the Epidemiologic Science" doi.org/10.1080/07315724.2014.992553

"Experimental Study of the Effects of Three Types of Meat on Endothelial Function in a Group of Healthy Volunteers" tinyurl.com/yyqmoaf6

"Meat subtypes and colorectal cancer risk: A pooled analysis of 6 cohort studies in Japan" doi.org/10.1111/cas.14188

"Processed and Unprocessed Red Meat and Risk of Colorectal Cancer: Analysis by Tumor Location and Modification by Time" doi.org/10.1371/journal.pone.0135959

"The role of red meat in the diet: nutrition and health benefits" doi.org/10.1017/S0029665115004267

"Nutritional labelling for promoting healthier food purchasing and consumption" tinyurl.com/y5wxhdy4

"Substitution of red meat with soybean but not non- soy legumes improves inflammation in patients with type 2 diabetes; a randomized clinical trial" ncbi.nlm.nih.gov/pmc/articles/PMC6405394/

"Effects of Total Red Meat Consumption on Glycemic Control and Inflammation: A Systematically Searched Meta-analysis and Meta-regression of Randomized Controlled Trials (OR22-08-19)" doi.org/10.1093/cdn/nzz028.OR22-08-19

"Isocaloric Diets High in Animal or Plant Protein Reduce Liver Fat and Inflammation in Individuals With Type 2 Diabetes" doi.org/10.1053/j.gastro.2016.10.007

"Consumption of a high-fat meal containing cheese compared with a vegan alternative lowers postprandial C-reactive protein in overweight and obese individuals with metabolic abnormalities: a randomised controlled cross-over study" doi.org/10.1017/jns.2015.40

"Potential effects of reduced red meat compared with increased fiber intake on glucose metabolism and liver fat content: a randomized and controlled dietary intervention study" doi.org/10.1093/ajcn/nqy307

"Whey protein lowers blood pressure and improves endothelial function and lipid biomarkers in adults with prehypertension and mild hypertension: results from the chronic Whey2Go randomized controlled trial" doi.org/10.3945/ajcn.116.137919

"Dietary Red and Processed Meat Intake and Markers of Adiposity and Inflammation: The Multiethnic Cohort Study" ncbi.nlm. nih.gov/pmc/articles/PMC5540319/

"Lean meat and heart health" pubmed.ncbi.nlm.nih.gov/15927927/

"Meat consumption and mortality - results from the European Prospective Investigation into Cancer and Nutrition" doi. org/10.1186/1741-7015-11-63

"Meat consumption and diet quality and mortality in NHANES III" doi.org/10.1038/ejcn.2013.59

"Beef in an Optimal Lean Diet study: effects on lipids, lipoproteins, and apolipoproteins" doi.org/10.3945/ajcn.111.016261

"Co-consumption of Vegetables and Fruit, Whole Grains, and Fiber Reduces the Cancer Risk of Red and Processed Meat in a Large Prospective Cohort of Adults from Alberta's Tomorrow Project" doi.org/10.3390/nu12082265

YOU DIDN'T REALLY COVER

"Negative, Null and Beneficial Effects of Drinking Water on Energy Intake, Energy Expenditure, Fat Oxidation and Weight Change in Randomized Trials: A Qualitative Review" doi.org/10.3390/nu8010019

"Water-Induced Thermogenesis" doi.org/10.1210/jc.2003-030780

See here for more info on hydration: tinyurl.com/y3b7tvh6

I HEAR DIET X IS

"Effects of a caloric restriction weight loss diet and exercise on inflammatory biomarkers in overweight/obese postmenopausal women: a randomized controlled trial" doi.org/10.1158/0008-5472.CAN-11-3092

"Low Carbohydrate versus Isoenergetic Balanced Diets for Reducing Weight and Cardiovascular Risk: A Systematic Review and Meta-Analysis" doi.org/10.1371/journal.pone.0100652

"Metabolic and behavioral effects of a high-sucrose diet during weight loss" doi.org/10.1093/ajcn/65.4.908

"Energy expenditure and body composition changes after an isocaloric ketogenic diet in overweight and obese men" doi. org/10.3945/ajcn.116.133561

"Effects of a Low–Glycemic Load vs Low-Fat Diet in Obese Young Adults" doi.org/10.1001/jama.297.19.2092

"Obesity Energetics: Body Weight Regulation and the Effects of Diet Composition" ncbi.nlm.nih.gov/pmc/articles/PMC5568065/

"Carbohydrate quantity in the dietary management of type 2 diabetes: A systematic review and meta-analysis" doi.org/10.1111/dom.13499

"Low Carbohydrate versus Isoenergetic Balanced Diets for Reducing Weight and Cardiovascular Risk: A Systematic Review and Meta-Analysis" doi.org/10.1371/journal.pone.0100652

"Effect of Alternate-Day Fasting on Weight Loss, Weight Maintenance, and Cardioprotection Among Metabolically Healthy Obese Adults" doi.org/10.1001/jamainternmed.2017.0936

"Efficacy of ketogenic diet on body composition during resistance training in trained men: a randomized controlled trial" doi. org/10.1186/s12970-018-0236-9

"Ketogenic low-carbohydrate diets have no metabolic advantage over nonketogenic low-carbohydrate diets" doi.org/10.1093/ajcn/83.5.1055

"Metabolic effects of very low calorie weight reduction diets" doi.org/10.1172/JCI111268

"Comparison of the Atkins, Ornish, Weight Watchers, and Zone Diets for Weight Loss and Heart Disease Risk Reduction" doi.org/10.1001/jama.293.1.43

"Effects of Low-Carbohydrate Diets Versus Low-Fat Diets on Metabolic Risk Factors: A Meta-Analysis of Randomized Controlled Clinical Trials" doi.org/10.1093/aje/kws264

"The BROAD study: A randomised controlled trial using a whole food plant-based diet in the community for obesity, ischaemic heart disease or diabetes" doi.org/10.1038/nutd.2017.3

"Long-Term Effects of 4 Popular Diets on Weight Loss and Cardiovascular Risk Factors" doi.org/10.1161/CIRCOUT-COMES.113.000723

"No Significant Effect of Dietary Carbohydrate versus Fat on the Reduction in Total Energy Expenditure During Maintenance of Lost Weight: A Secondary Analysis" doi.org/10.1101/476655

"Comparison of Nutritional Quality of the Vegan, Vegetarian, Semi-Vegetarian, Pesco-Vegetarian and Omnivorous Diet" doi.org/10.3390/nu6031318

"Effects of a DASH-like diet containing lean beef onvascular health" doi.org/10.1038/jhh.2014.34

"Dietary modifications for weight loss and weight loss maintenance" doi.org/10.1016/j.metabol.2019.01.001

"The Mediterranean Diet and Cardiovascular Health" doi.org/10.1161/CIRCRESAHA.118.313348

"Dietary habits and mortality in 11,000 vegetarians and health conscious people: results of a 17 year follow up" doi.org/10.1136/bmj.313.7060.775

"Vegetarian diet and all-cause mortality: Evidence from a large population-based Australian cohort - the 45 and Up Study" pubmed.ncbi.nlm.nih.gov/28040519/

REFERENCES

"Adipokines – removing road blocks to obesity and diabetes therapy" ncbi.nlm.nih.gov/pmc/articles/PMC3986498/

"Adipokines in health and disease" doi.org/10.1016/j.tips.2015.04.014

"Mortality in vegetarians and comparable nonvegetarians in the United Kingdom" doi.org/10.3945/ajcn.115.119461

"Effects of Time-Restricted Eating on Weight Loss and Other Metabolic Parameters in Women and Men With Overweight and Obesity" doi.org/10.1001/jamainternmed.2020.4153

"Being cool: how body temperature influences ageing and longevity" doi.org/10.1007/s10522-015-9571-2

"Lifespan - Why We Age And Why We Don't Have To" - Simon & Schuster, Inc. (2019). David A. Sinclair.

"Exercise Prevents Diet-Induced Cellular Senescence in Adipose Tissue" doi.org/10.2337/db15-0291

"Physical Exercise Prevents Cellular Senescence in Circulating Leukocytes and in the Vessel Wall" doi.org/10.1161/CIRCULATIONAHA.109.861005

SO A CALORIE IS A CALORIE

"Trans-Fats and Coronary Heart Disease" doi.org/10.1080/10408398.2010.526872

ARE YOU REALLY TELLING ME I DON'T HAVE TO COUNT CALORIES?

"Objective versus Self-Reported Energy Intake Changes During Low-Carbohydrate and Low-Fat Diets" doi.org/10.1002/oby.22389

"Discrepancy between Self-Reported and Actual Caloric Intake and Exercise in Obese Subjects" doi.org/10.1056/NEJM199212313272701

"Evaluation of dietary assessment instruments against doubly labeled water, a biomarker of habitual energy intake" doi.org/10.1152/ajpendo.2001.281.5.E891

"Prevalence and characteristics of misreporting of energy intake in US adults: NHANES 2003–2012" doi.org/10.1017/S0007114515002706

"Intentional mis-reporting of food consumption and its relationship with body mass index and psychological scores in women" doi.org/10.1111/j.1365-277X.2004.00520.x

"Energy Intake and Energy Expenditure" doi.org/10.1016/S0002-8223(02)90316-0

"Accuracy in Wrist-Worn, Sensor-Based Measurements of Heart Rate and Energy Expenditure in a Diverse Cohort" doi.org/10.3390/jpm7020003

"Calorie counting and fitness tracking technology: Associations with eating disorder symptomatology" doi.org/10.1016/j.eatbeh.2017.02.002

"My fitness pal usage in men: Associations with eating disorder symptoms and psychosocial impairment" doi.org/10.1016/j.eatbeh.2019.02.003

"My Fitness Pal Calorie Tracker Usage in the Eating Disorders" ncbi.nlm.nih.gov/pmc/articles/PMC5700836/

"Eating Slowly Increases the Postprandial Response of the Anorexigenic Gut Hormones, Peptide YY and Glucagon-Like Peptide-1" doi.org/10.1210/jc.2009-1018

"A systematic review and meta-analysis examining the effect of eating rate on energy intake and hunger" doi.org/10.3945/ajcn.113.081745

"Effects of changes in eating speed on obesity in patients with diabetes: a secondary analysis of longitudinal health check-up data" dx.doi.org/10.1136/bmjopen-2017-019589

"Rigid dietary control, flexible dietary control, and intuitive eating: Evidence for their differential relationship to disordered eating and body image concerns" pubmed.ncbi.nlm.nih.gov/28131005/

"Flexible Eating Behavior Predicts Greater Weight Loss Following a Diet and Exercise Intervention in Older Women" doi.org/10.1080/21551197.2018.1435433

"Helpful or harmful? The comparative value of self-weighing and calorie counting versus intuitive eating on the eating disorder symptomology of college students" doi.org/10.1007/s40519-018-0562-6

"A Health at Every Size intervention improves intuitive eating and diet quality in Canadian women" doi.org/10.1016/j.clnu.2016.06.008

"Can patients with eating disorders learn to eat intuitively? A 2-year pilot study" doi.org/10.1080/10640266.2017.1279907

"Psychological flexibility mediates change in intuitive eating regulation in acceptance and commitment therapy interventions" doi.org/10.1017/S1368980017000441

"A structured literature review on the role of mindfulness, mindful eating and intuitive eating in changing eating behaviours: effectiveness and associated potential mechanisms" doi.org/10.1017/S0954422417000154

"Mindfulness Approaches and Weight Loss, Weight Maintenance, and Weight Regain" doi.org/10.1007/s13679-018-0299-6

FIBRE BLOATS AND MAKES ME FEEL WEIRD

"Effects of Gut Microbes on Nutrient Absorption and Energy Regulation" ncbi.nlm.nih.gov/pmc/articles/PMC3601187/

"Linking Long-Term Dietary Patterns with Gut Microbial Enterotypes" ncbi.nlm.nih.gov/pmc/articles/PMC3368382/

115

BEAT YOUR WEIGHT BEAT YOUR FAT

I WANT TO CONTINUE TO EAT

"No Effect of Added Sugar Consumed at Median American Intake Level on Glucose Tolerance or Insulin Resistance" doi.org/10.3390/nu7105430

"Relationship between Added Sugars Consumption and Chronic Disease Risk Factors: Current Understanding" doi.org/10.3390/nu8110697

"Controversies about sugars: results from systematic reviews and meta-analyses on obesity, cardiometabolic disease and diabetes" doi.org/10.1007/s00394-016-1345-3

"Dietary sugars and cardiometabolic risk: systematic review and meta-analyses of randomized controlled trials of the effects on blood pressure and lipids" doi.org/10.3945/ajcn.113.081521

"Effects of free sugars on blood pressure and lipids: a systematic review and meta-analysis of nutritional isoenergetic intervention trials" doi.org/10.3945/ajcn.116.139253

"Reducing free sugars intake in adults to reduce the risk of noncommunicable diseases" tinyurl.com/y2w5lufv

WHAT ABOUT CHEAT MEALS?

"The runaway weight gain train: too many accelerators, not enough brakes" doi.org/10.1136/bmj.329.7468.736

"Role of leptin in the neuroendocrine response to fasting" doi.org/10.1038/382250a0

"Leptin Not Impressive in Clinical Trial" doi.org/10.1126/science.286.5441.881a

"How Fat Works" - Harvard University Press (2009). Philip A. Wood

"Effects of Recombinant Leptin Therapy in a Child with Congenital Leptin Deficiency" doi.org/10.1056/NEJM199909163411204

CAN I TARGET FAT LOSS?

There's been quite a bit of work done in the area of spot reduction and the vast majority of studies show that it's not a thing.

"The effect of abdominal exercise on abdominal fat" doi.org/10.1519/JSC.0b013e3181fb4a46

"Subcutaneous Fat Alterations Resulting from an Upper-Body Resistance Training Program" doi.org/10.1249/mss.0b0138058a5cb

"Effects of Sit up Exercise Training on Adipose Cell Size and Adiposity" doi.org/10.1080/02701367.1984.10609359

WHAT TO DO ABOUT HUNGER?

"The effect of caffeine on energy balance" doi.org/10.1515/jbcpp-2016-0090

"Dairy products, satiety and food intake: A meta-analysis of clinical trials" doi.org/10.1016/j.clnu.2016.01.017

"Activation of temperature-sensitive TRPV1-like receptors in ARC POMC neurons reduces food intake" doi.org/10.1371/journal.pbio.2004399

"Sleep influences on obesity, insulin resistance, and risk of type 2 diabetes" doi.org/10.1016/j.metabol.2018.02.010

"Association of sleep disturbances with obesity, insulin resistance and the metabolic syndrome" doi.org/10.1016/j.metabol.2018.04.001

GENES OR ENVIRONMENT?

"The Evolution of Obesity" - Johns Hopkins University Press (2009). Michael L. Power, Jay Schulkin

"Human Energy Requirements: A Manual for Planners and Nutritionists" doi.org/10.1093/ajcn/53.6.1506

"The thrifty phenotype: An adaptation in growth or metabolism?" doi.org/10.1002/ajhb.21100

"Epidemiology, genes and the environment: lessons learned from the Helsinki Birth Cohort Study" doi.org/10.1111/j.1365-2796.2007.01798.x

"The genetic contribution to non-syndromic human obesity" doi.org/10.1038/nrg2594

"Metabolic Syndrome: Genetic Insights into Disease Pathogenesis" ncbi.nlm.nih.gov/pmc/articles/PMC5141383/

"Genetic variants and the metabolic syndrome: a systematic review" doi.org/10.1111/j.1467-789X.2011.00907.x

"A Twin Study of Human Obesity" doi.org/10.1001/jama.1986.03380010055024

"The Body-Mass Index of Twins Who Have Been Reared Apart" doi.org/10.1056/NEJM199005243222102

"High-Risk Populations: The Pimas of Arizona and Mexico" ncbi.nlm.nih.gov/pmc/articles/PMC4418458/

"Multiplex Genome Engineering Using CRISPR/Cas Systems" ncbi.nlm.nih.gov/pmc/articles/PMC3795411/

"Physical Activity and the Association of Common FTO Gene Variants With Body Mass Index and Obesity" doi.org/10.1001/archinte.168.16.1791

WHAT ABOUT THE MICROBIOME?

"Evolution in Health and Disease" - Oxford University Press (2007). Stephen C. Stearns and Jacob C. Koella

"The Human Gut Microbiome and Body Metabolism: Implications for Obesity and Diabetes" doi.org/10.1373/clinchem.2012.187617

REFERENCES

"Obesity and the gut microbiome: Striving for causality" doi.org/10.1016/j.molmet.2012.07.002

"Influence of Gut Microbiota on Subclinical Inflammation and Insulin Resistance" doi.org/10.1155/2013/986734

"Gut Microbiome and Obesity: A Plausible Explanation for Obesity" ncbi.nlm.nih.gov/pmc/articles/PMC4443745/

"Evaluating Causality of Gut Microbiota in Obesity and Diabetes in Humans" doi.org/10.1210/er.2017-00192

"Effects of perinatal exposure to palatable diets on body weight and sensitivity to drugs of abuse in rats" tinyurl.com/yxpl98fq

"The thrifty phenotype hypothesis: Type 2 diabetes" doi.org/10.1093/bmb/60.1.5

"Adolescent Fiber Consumption Is Associated with Visceral Fat and Inflammatory Markers" doi.org/10.1210/jc.2012-1784

"Probiotics, their health benefits and applications for developing healthier foods: a review" doi.org/10.1111/j.1574-6968.2012.02593.x

"Health benefits and practical aspects of high-fiber diets" doi.org/10.1093/ajcn/59.5.1242S

"Effect on Blood Lipids of Very High Intakes of Fiber in Diets Low in Saturated Fat and Cholesterol" doi.org/10.1056/NEJM199307013290104

"Impact of Dietary Fiber Consumption on Insulin Resistance and the Prevention of Type 2 Diabetes" doi.org/10.1093/jn/nxx008

"Dietary Fiber and Telomere Length in 5674 U.S. Adults: An NHANES Study of Biological Aging" doi.org/10.3390/nu10040400

"What Do We Know about Dietary Fiber Intake in Children and Health? The Effects of Fiber Intake on Constipation, Obesity, and Diabetes in Children" doi.org/10.3945/an.111.001362

"Cereal fibre intake and risk of mortality from all causes, CVD, cancer and inflammatory diseases: a systematic review and meta-analysis of prospective cohort studies" doi.org/10.1017/S0007114516001938

"Dietary fibre and incidence of type 2 diabetes in eight European countries: the EPIC-InterAct Study and a meta-analysis of prospective studies" dx.doi.org/10.1007%2Fs00125-015-3585-9

"Dietary fiber intake, dietary glycemic index and load, and body mass index" doi.org/10.1038/sj.ejcn.1602610

WHAT ABOUT ANTIBIOTICS?

"The core gut microbiome, energy balance and obesity" doi.org/10.1113/jphysiol.2009.174136

"Long-term impacts of antibiotic exposure on the human intestinal microbiota" doi.org/10.1099/mic.0.040618-0

"Cesarean section and risk of obesity in childhood, adolescence, and early adulthood: evidence from 3 Brazilian birth cohorts" doi.org/10.3945/ajcn.111.026401

"Altering the intestinal microbiota during a critical developmental window has lasting metabolic consequences" doi.org/10.1016/j.cell.2014.05.052

"Gut microbiota of healthy Canadian infants: profiles by mode of delivery and infant diet at 4 months" doi.org/10.1503/cmaj.121189

"The Risks of Not Breastfeeding for Mothers and Infants" ncbi.nlm.nih.gov/pmc/articles/PMC2812877/

"Many ways to die, one way to arrive: how selection acts through pregnancy" doi.org/10.1016/j.tig.2013.03.001

WOMEN?

"Ancient Bodies, Modern Lives: How Evolution Has Shaped Women's Health" - OUP USA (2010). Wenda Trevathan

"On Fertile Ground - A Natural History of Human Reproduction" - Harvard University Press (2003). Peter T. Ellison

"Sex Differences in Energy Metabolism Need to Be Considered with Lifestyle Modifications in Humans" doi.org/10.1155/2011/391809

"How Fat Works" Harvard University Press (2009). Philip A. Wood

"Sex Differences in Exercise Metabolism and the Role of 17-Beta Estradiol" doi.org/10.1249/MSS.0b013e31816212ff

"Comparative and Evolutionary Dimensions of the Energetics of Human Pregnancy and Lactation" tinyurl.com/y34yy3q2

"Primate Milk: Proximate Mechanisms and Ultimate Perspectives" tinyurl.com/y4yq2lms

"Nutrition Recommendations in Pregnancy and Lactation" ncbi.nlm.nih.gov/pmc/articles/PMC5104202/

"The Normal Menstrual Cycle and the Control of Ovulation" ncbi.nlm.nih.gov/books/NBK279054/

"Regulation of energy expenditure by estradiol in premenopausal women" doi.org/10.1152/japplphysiol.00473.2015

"Response to resistance training in young women and men" pubmed.ncbi.nlm.nih.gov/7558529/

"Resistance Training Combined With Diet Decreases Body Fat While Preserving Lean Mass Independent of Resting Metabolic Rate: A Randomized Trial" tinyurl.com/y6f2rf6y

"Technical guidance on nutrition labelling" tinyurl.com/ycq7rog3

"Food information to consumers - legislation" ec.europa.eu/food/safety/labelling_nutrition/labelling_legislation_en

"REGULATION (EU)... on the provision of food information to consumers..." eur-lex.europa.eu/LexUriServ/LexUriServ.do?uri=OJ:L:2011:304:0018:0063:EN:PDF

"Guidance for Industry: Guide for Developing and Using Data Bases for Nutrition Labeling" tinyurl.com/y3zkkb97

APPENDIX 2 - HOW TO READ NUTRITION LABELS

(UK) "Technical guidance on nutrition labelling" tinyurl.com/ycq7rog3

(EU) "REGULATION (EU)... on the provision of food information to consumers..." tinyurl.com/y46z5gat

(US) "Guidance for Industry: Guide for Developing and Using Data Bases for Nutrition Labeling" tinyurl.com/y3zkkb97

APPENDIX 5 - HOW TO EAT HEALTHY WHEN MONEY IS TIGHT

"Examining the interaction of fast-food outlet exposure and income on diet and obesity: evidence from 51,361 UK Biobank participants" doi.org/10.1186/s12966-018-0699-8

"Does neighborhood fast-food outlet exposure amplify inequalities in diet and obesity? A cross-sectional study" doi.org/10.3945/ajcn.115.128132

"Are exposures to ready-to-eat food environments associated with type 2 diabetes? A cross-sectional study of 347 551 UK Biobank adult participants" doi.org/10.1016/S2542-5196(18)30208-0

APPENDIX 6 - INSULIN SENSITIVITY

"Impact of Brain Insulin Signaling on Dopamine Function, Food Intake, Reward, and Emotional Behavior" pubmed.ncbi.nlm.nih.gov/31001792/

"Low-Fat Versus Low-Carbohydrate Weight Reduction Diets: Effects on Weight Loss, Insulin Resistance, and Cardiovascular Risk: A Randomized Control Trial" doi.org/10.2337/db09-0098

"A Single Night of Partial Sleep Deprivation Induces Insulin Resistance in Multiple Metabolic Pathways in Healthy Subjects" doi.org/10.1210/jc.2009-2430

"Sleep characteristics and insulin sensitivity in humans" pubmed.ncbi.nlm.nih.gov/25248582/

"Chromium and polyphenols from cinnamon improve insulin sensitivity: Plenary Lecture" doi.org/10.1017/S0029665108006010

"Cinnamon: Potential Role in the Prevention of Insulin Resistance, Metabolic Syndrome, and Type 2 Diabetes" doi.org/10.1177%2F193229681000400324

"Reduction in Added Sugar Intake and Improvement in Insulin Secretion in Overweight Latina Adolescents" ncbi.nlm.nih.gov/pmc/articles/PMC2847394/

"The Role of Carbohydrates in Insulin Resistance" doi.org/10.1093/jn/131.10.2782S

"Strength training improves muscle quality and insulin sensitivity in Hispanic older adults with type 2 diabetes" doi.org/10.7150/ijms.4.19

"Exercise Training and Insulin Resistance: A Current Review" dx.doi.org/10.4172%2F2165-7904.S5-003

"The effects of aerobic, resistance, and combination training on insulin sensitivity and secretion in overweight adults" pubmed.ncbi.nlm.nih.gov/25882384/

"Both resistance- and endurance-type exercise reduce the prevalence of hyperglycaemia in individuals with impaired glucose tolerance and in insulin-treated and non-insulin-treated type 2 diabetic patients" doi.org/10.1007/s00125-011-2380-5

"Dietary fibre consumption and insulin resistance – the role of body fat and physical activity" doi.org/10.1017/S0007114512004953

"Effects of ginger (Zingiber officinale) on plasma glucose level, HbA1c and insulin sensitivity in type 2 diabetic patients" doi.org/10.3109/09637486.2013.775223

"Effect of green tea on glucose control and insulin sensitivity: a meta-analysis of 17 randomized controlled trials" doi.org/10.3945/ajcn.112.052746

"Effects of Green Tea Extract on Insulin Resistance and Glucagon-Like Peptide 1 in Patients with Type 2 Diabetes and Lipid Abnormalities: A Randomized, Double-Blinded, and Placebo-Controlled Trial" ncbi.nlm.nih.gov/pmc/articles/PMC3948786/

"The role of fatty acids in insulin resistance" doi.org/10.1186/s12944-015-0123-1

"Effect of magnesium supplementation on insulin resistance in humans: A systematic review" doi.org/10.1016/j.nut.2017.01.009

"Effects of Saturated Fat, Polyunsaturated Fat, Monounsaturated Fat, and Carbohydrate on Glucose-Insulin Homeostasis: A Systematic Review and Meta-analysis of Randomised Controlled Feeding Trials" doi.org/10.1371/journal.pmed.1002087

"The Effects of Mental Stress on Non-insulin-dependent Diabetes: Determining the Relationship Between Catecholamine and Adrenergic Signals from Stress, Anxiety, and Depression on the Physiological Changes in the Pancreatic Hormone Secretion" doi.org/10.7759/cureus.5474

"A Single Night of Partial Sleep Deprivation Induces Insulin Resistance in Multiple Metabolic Pathways in Healthy Subjects" doi.org/10.1210/jc.2009-2430

"Sleep characteristics and insulin sensitivity in humans" pubmed.ncbi.nlm.nih.gov/25248582/

"Association of sleep disturbances with obesity, insulin resistance and the metabolic syndrome" doi.org/10.1016/j.metabol.2018.04.001

REFERENCES

"Beneficial Impact of Sleep Extension on Fasting Insulin Sensitivity in Adults with Habitual Sleep Restriction" doi.org/10.5665/sleep.4660

"Vinegar Improves Insulin Sensitivity to a High-Carbohydrate Meal in Subjects With Insulin Resistance or Type 2 Diabetes" doi.org/10.2337/diacare.27.1.281

"Vinegar Consumption Increases Insulin-Stimulated Glucose Uptake by the Forearm Muscle in Humans with Type 2 Diabetes" doi.org/10.1155/2015/175204

APPENDIX 7 - FOOD

"Determination Of Energy Values For Fibers" ncbi.nlm.nih.gov/books/NBK223593/

"Pathways to obesity" doi.org/10.1038/sj.ijo.0802123

MAIN INGREDIENTS

Energy values can be all over the place, depending on whether you look it up, calculate it yourself, or use general or specific factors (as well as cooked or uncooked, with cooking generally increasing available calories, sometimes considerably, e.g. potatoes, due to breaking down the cells, which increases the bioavailability). In the end I settled on uncooked averages from the following 4 sites (gross outliers were removed from the averaging), so calories given are basically an averaging of the general (Atwater) and specific (Atwater correction) factors:

ars.usda.gov/northeast-area/beltsville-md-bhnrc/beltsville-human-nutrition-research-center/food-surveys-research-group/docs/fndds-download-databases/ (Ingredient Nutrient Values)

nutritionix.com/database

nutritiondata.self.com/

fatsecret.com/calories-nutrition/

TO BOOST HDL

"Dietary unsaturated fat increases HDL metabolic pathways involving apoE favorable to reverse cholesterol transport" doi.org/10.1172/jci.insight.124620

"Chronic consumption of a low calorie, high polyphenol cranberry beverage attenuates inflammation and improves glucoregulation and HDL cholesterol in healthy overweight humans: a randomized controlled trial" doi.org/10.1007/s00394-018-1643-z

"Health effects of trans-fatty acids: experimental and observational evidence" doi.org/10.1038/sj.ejcn.1602973

"Changes in markers for cardio-metabolic disease risk after only 1-2 weeks of a high saturated fat diet in overweight adults" doi.org/10.1371/journal.pone.0198372

"Blood Lipid and Lipoprotein Adaptations to Exercise" doi.org/10.2165/00007256-200131150-00002

BIOTICS

"Dietary intake and cognitive function: evidence from the Bogalusa Heart Study" ncbi.nlm.nih.gov/pmc/articles/PMC6900495/

"Preventing dementia: do vitamin and mineral supplements have a role?" cochrane.org/news/preventing-dementia-do-vitamin-and-mineral-supplements-have-role

"Vegetarian Diets and Blood Pressure A Meta-analysis" doi.org/10.1001/jamainternmed.2013.14547

"Fruit and vegetable consumption and breast cancer incidence: Repeated measures over 30 years of follow-up" doi.org/10.1002/ijc.31653

"Fruit and vegetable consumption and mortality from all causes, cardiovascular disease, and cancer: systematic review and dose-response meta-analysis of prospective cohort studies" doi.org/10.1136/bmj.g4490

"Fruit and Vegetable Intake and Risk of Major Chronic Disease" doi.org/10.1093/jnci/djh296

"Fruit and vegetable consumption and stroke: meta-analysis of cohort studies" doi.org/10.1016/S0140-6736(06)68069-0

Biotics and the microbiome is a rapidly moving and expanding field and is practically impossible to try and stay abreast of.

"The Host Microbiome Regulates and Maintains Human Health: A Primer and Perspective for Non-Microbiologists" doi.org/10.1158/0008-5472.CAN-16-2929

"Integrative medicine and human health - the role of pre-, pro- and synbiotics" doi.org/10.1186/2001-1326-1-6

"The role of short chain fatty acids in appetite regulation and energy homeostasis" doi.org/10.1038/ijo.2015.84

"Gut microbiota as a regulator of energy homeostasis and ectopic fat deposition: mechanisms and implications for metabolic disorders" doi.org/10.1097/MOL.0b013e3283347ebb

"Interaction between microbiota and immunity in health and disease" doi.org/10.1038/s41422-020-0332-7

"Microbiome definition re-visited: old concepts and new challenges" doi.org/10.1186/s40168-020-00875-0

"Potential Health Benefits of Olive Oil and Plant Polyphenols" doi.org/10.3390/ijms19030686

"Novel insights of dietary polyphenols and obesity" doi.org/10.1016/j.jnutbio.2013.09.001

"Benefits of polyphenols on gut microbiota and implications in human health" doi.org/10.1016/j.jnutbio.2013.05.001

"Chronic consumption of a low calorie, high polyphenol cranberry beverage attenuates inflammation and improves glucoregulation and HDL cholesterol in healthy overweight humans: a randomized controlled trial" doi.org/10.1007/s00394-018-1643-z

"Biological Relevance of Extra Virgin Olive Oil Polyphenols Metabolites" doi.org/10.3390/antiox7120170

"The role of Gut Microbiota in the development of obesity and Diabetes" doi.org/10.1186/s12944-016-0278-4

"Gut microbiota composition correlates with diet and health in the elderly" doi.org/10.1038/nature11319

"Probiotics and their Effects on Metabolic Diseases: An Update" doi.org/10.7860/JCDR/2012/5004.2701

"Reduction in the Incidence of Type 2 Diabetes with Lifestyle Intervention or Metformin" doi.org/10.1056/NEJMoa012512

"The role of microbes and autoimmunity in the pathogenesis of neuropsychiatric illness" doi.org/10.1097/BOR.0b013e32836208de

"Melancholic microbes: a link between gut microbiota and depression?" doi.org/10.1111/nmo.12198

"Brain-Gut Interactions in Inflammatory Bowel Disease" doi.org/10.1053/j.gastro.2012.10.003

Printed in Poland
by Amazon Fulfillment
Poland Sp. z o.o., Wrocław